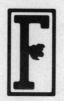

Making Sense of Menopause

Over 150 Women and Experts
Share Their Wisdom, Experience, and
Commonsense Advice

FAYE KITCHENER CONE

A FIRESIDE BOOK
Published by Simon & Schuster
New York   London   Toronto   Sydney   Tokyo   Singapore

FIRESIDE

Rockefeller Center
1230 Avenue of the Americas
New York, New York 10020

Copyright © 1993 by Faye Kitchener Cone

FIRESIDE and colophon are registered trademarks
of Simon & Schuster Inc.

Designed by Marysarah Quinn
Manufactured in the United States of America

10   9

Library of Congress Cataloging-in-Publication Data

Cone, Faye Kitchener.
    Making sense of menopause : over 150 women and experts share their
wisdom, experience, and commonsense advice / Faye
Kitchener Cone.
        p.   cm.
    "A Fireside book."
    Includes index.
    1. Menopause—Popular works.   I. Title.
RG186.C627   1993
618.1'75—dc20   93-2526   CIP
ISBN 0-671-78638-5

The ideas, procedures, and suggestions in this book are intended
to supplement, not replace, the medical advice of trained
professionals. All matters regarding your health require medical
supervision. Consult your physician before adopting the medical
suggestions in this book, as well as about any condition that
may require diagnosis or medical attention.

The authors and publishers disclaim any liability arising
directly or indirectly from the use of this book.

Acknowledgments

Until I became a writer, my success in advertising was always based on the collaborative process that is key to good marketing and communication. What a surprise it was to find myself alone with a word processor, research notes, and a telephone—it was clear that I would have to produce this book all by myself. Now that it's complete, it was more of a team effort than I had anticipated. Without help from the following people, it never would have been written.

Friends always come first and I have been lucky to receive endless support, but several deserve to be singled out, in particular: Dr. Mardy Grothe, psychologist, who provided the encouragement I needed to embark on this project; Tom Teicholz, author and self-proclaimed manager of my literary career, who helped me find my way through the publishing world and spent many hours counseling, reviewing the manuscript, dispensing valuable advice, and being a good friend; Lexy Tanner, vice president at Chiat/Day Advertising, who helped get the first focus research groups off the ground; Linda Gay Blanc, formerly executive vice president of Burson-Marstellar, who shared her Rolodex and rounded up dozens of wonderful women for me to interview; Holly Buskirk, who acted as head cheerleader as we burned up the telephone lines between New York and Dallas, provided another viewpoint, put together a unique focus group of very special women, and remained my strongest supporter throughout this project; and Mary and Dick Auletta, who separately and together were there to help out in any way possible.

A special note of gratitude goes to the following doctors and health professionals who took more than a passing interest in my work, provided lengthy interviews, and spent extra time to carefully review the manuscript for accuracy: at New York's Hospital for Special Surgery, Dr. Richard Bockman, chief of endocrinology, and Theresa Galsworthy, R.N., director of the Osteoporosis Center; at Memorial Sloan-Kettering Cancer Center, Dr. Daiva Bajrounas and Dr. Jamie Ostroff; Dr. James Simon, chief of reproductive endocrinology at Georgetown University Medical Center; Dr. Elizabeth Lee Vliet, medical director, Elizabeth Paul Center, and women's health consultant, Canyon Ranch; Dr. Serafina Corsello; Dr. Leo Galland; and Dr. Judyth Reichenberg-Ullman.

Without a medical background, I relied heavily on many health professionals to sort out often confusing information and put it together in a way that would make sense to the layperson. The following doctors gave generously of their time: Dr. Amy Altenhaus, Dr. Alan Altman, Dr. Joseph Bark, Dr. Steven Bock, Dr. Fran Ginsberg, Dr. Charles Hammond, Dr. William Hoskins, Dr. Valerie Jorgensen, Dr. Albert Kligman, Dr. Fredi Kronenberg, Dr. Hank Liers, Dr. Phyllis Mansfield, Dr. Bruce Patsner, Dr. Veronica Ravnikar, Dr. Quentin Regestein, and Dr. Jing Nuan Wu.

Thanks also go to Janine O'Leary Cobb, editor of A Friend Indeed; Monica Miller, health care advocate and director of the People's Consortium for Medical Freedom; and Kate Ruddon of the American College of Obstetrics and Gynecology, who helped guide me in my research and supplied valuable contacts and resources.

Undoubtedly, asking someone close to you to read a manuscript is a real test of friendship, passed with flying colors by the following people, to whom I am enormously grateful: Alice Goodman, Eve Luppert, Sharon Medford, Sheila O'Brien, and Janice Papolos.

None of this would have happened without the help and encouragement of my agent, Emilie Jacobson, whose no-nonsense approach to getting things done kept me on track. Sydny Miner, executive editor at Simon & Schuster, definitely made this book better with her careful guidance and rigorous scrutiny. Both Nancy Monson, who came to the research rescue when I needed her most and also painstakingly reviewed parts of the manuscript, and Betty Shaughnessy, who transcribed hundreds of interviews, were reliable collaborators in this effort.

Finally, my greatest debt of gratitude goes to the hundreds of women who gave deeply and shared some of their most intimate thoughts. I would often finish an interview, put down the telephone, and think about how lucky I was to know some of these women, even fleetingly. Their stories are what makes this book special and I thank them with all my heart.

Boston
January 1993

To Steve, and to Cliff

Contents

Introduction

When I was a young girl, I didn't know what every young girl should know. Now I'm going to be an old lady, and I don't even know what every old lady should know.
— Edith Bunker, "Edith's Problem,"
All in the Family

Four summers ago I spent a week in Aspen with one of my best friends. The days were sunny and warm and the evenings refreshingly cool, just as they should be in the mountains. We shared a room and slept with the windows open. One night I awoke around 3:00 A.M. and couldn't understand why the room was so warm; I slept with the covers off for the rest of the night.

When I remarked to my friend in the morning about the sudden heat during the night, she looked at me strangely and said she hadn't noticed the change. It took a few more nights of the same and some serious detective work before I realized what had happened—I'd had my first hot flash.

That was when I was 42. My mother hadn't told me much about menopause, and Edith Bunker and her family weren't around anymore. What was happening to me and how was I supposed to figure out what to do about it?

Being an educated, take-charge individual, I was not about to be left in the dark about this major physical phenomenon. I canvassed bookstores, libraries, and shelves of periodicals and talked to my doctor, friends, and my mother to learn about menopause. To my surprise, menopause was not only a complex subject but also a controversial one. What's more, I discovered that very few women knew much about it and, in fact, were anxious and fearful of becoming menopausal.

The time seemed ripe to clear the air, get the facts straight, and put menopause in a modern perspective. Coincidentally, I was in the middle of a career transition—moving from eighteen years in the advertising world to writing nonfiction—and decided to combine these two life events: learn everything there was to know about menopause and create a readable book on the subject for other women.

What This Book Is About

Making Sense of Menopause is first and foremost a guidebook. It is filled with the most current information available on menopause, presented in an easy-to-read format. Each chapter is outlined in detail in the table of contents so you will be able to quickly find what you're looking for. There are guides that separate the known facts from those in question and sample charts to use to track your progression through the menopausal years. From information about menopause clinics to specifics on bone density measurement for osteoporosis, you will find practical information at your fingertips to help with day-to-day midlife issues.

Second, this book is unbiased and presents all sides of the menopause story. Controversial topics like hormone replacement therapy are presented in a balanced way so that you will have the facts at hand and be able to make your own decision. Alternative treatments for menopause are also discussed in detail and may offer new and less controversial options. If there is any bias in this book, it is my personal conviction that women must take a greater role in their own health care. Throughout these pages, you will find ways to cope with and take control of your menopause experience.

Third, this is the heart-to-heart talk you never had with your mother. You will be able to listen to the clear voices of hundreds of women who share their midlife common sense and wisdom about menopause. In their own words, they tell you how they talked to their partners, coped with the fear and uncertainty of what was happening to them, controlled their emotions, and made changes in their lives. These are women who eventually took charge of their situations and handled them with a positive view toward the future. Career women. Mothers. Single women. Grandmothers. Divorced women. Gay women. Childless women.

How This Book Was Put Together

Not easily, is the truth of it. Instead of an inspiring muse, I had an annoying little voice next to my ear that kept this book on track. This voice was the composite of many women's constant questions—the ones you are always afraid to ask your doctor or even your best friend, the ones that sound stupid but are critical in getting through the next day.

Not being part of the medical community also turned out to be a benefit. Although this made work more difficult on a day-to-day basis, it also allowed me to represent the majority of women who need to get the answers to their questions in terms they can understand, with no medical jargon. I often felt like an envoy in talking with doctors, psychologists, and epidemiologists. It was a terrific position to be in—I could probe and probe and probe until I had an answer that made sense to me and, by extension, to other women.

In an effort to better understand the scope of menopause issues facing women at midlife, I conducted four focus groups in New York, Connecticut, Boston, and Dallas and spoke to numerous individuals throughout the country as well. No matter whether the women had already experienced menopause or were fearfully anticipating its arrival, all echoed a single theme—ignorance. One woman expressed her frustration with her lack of knowledge by blaming other women for not sharing, especially mothers.

I asked my mother, "What did you know about menopause from your mother?"

"Nothing," she replied.

"You mean your mother went through it and she didn't tell you what it would be like?"

Isn't that incredible? She went through it, her mother went through it, her mother's mother went through it, we're all going to go through it—talk about a collective experience. And we still don't know anything!

Single woman, 48

To remedy this situation, I relied heavily on the medical and research communities for the facts and turned to women and sometimes men to ferret out the real-life solutions to menopause-related problems. Doctors went out of their way to make sure I expressed the medical facts correctly. Women gave unselfishly to help other women get through a similar experience.

Over a ten-month period, I interviewed more than 150 women over the telephone. Perhaps it was the guarantee of anonymity or the sense of intimacy conveyed by the telephone that encouraged these women to speak candidly and from the heart. Whatever the reason, their stories, which appear throughout the book, help convey what menopause is really all about. One of these women wrote me a thank-you note in which she talked about the changes wrought by menopause. It's a very personal reflection, but one that is shared by many women.

I know you're protecting my identity, but I'm not sure "Single mother, 58" describes who I am now. While my primary and most important goal in life was to have at least four or more children and be the best mother I could be (and to my great and everlasting satisfaction I did achieve that), all of my children are grown and independent now. I remember dreading this time. Despite the fact that I always worked, at least part-time, I used to think that nothing could ever compete with motherhood. And I wondered how I would ever find a different identity once my children were grown.

But I think that our lives are composed of chapters. Just as each stage of our children's lives brings us pleasures we couldn't have imagined, each stage of our own lives, if we are open to them, brings us great pleasure, too. Now I get a chance to discover different facets of myself. It's a heady experience. I turned out to be much broader and more competent than I ever thought I could be. If mothering is part of my current life, it is really grandmothering that takes up most of my nurturing time. My major activity is my work as a registered nurse and case manager for 120 clients receiving health care in their homes. I teach, I have a social life, I counsel, I am a part-time university student, and I write. I'm good at these things. I love them. I make a difference in my part of the world. It doesn't matter a lot to me how you refer to me, but now I am more than my motherhood.

What This Book Can Do for You

If you are interested in knowing what to expect during menopause and have a curiosity about what lies beyond, you will find solid answers to your questions. There is enough information in the following pages to help determine what is relevant to you, steer you in the direction of additional data, and expedite decision making about your long-term health.

Menopause is not a disease, nor is it the symbol of old age. By the time you finish this book, there is a good chance that you will have gained a positive attitude about this life transition, grown from the shared experiences of other women, and developed a sense of optimism about the future.

Chapter One

Are You Going Through Menopause?

Menopause—the last taboo, the final frontier. Menopause, where, for sure, no man has ever gone before. Menopause with all its mystery and unanswered questions: Is it really happening to me? Can I avoid it completely? Is it as bad as everyone says? At 44, aren't I too young?

Well, it is time to drop the drama. Menopause is a natural physical transition experienced by all women who exist past the age of 50. They all live to tell the story. Without a doubt, you will find menopause to be new, different, perhaps an adventure, and even challenging. Most of all, menopause will be yet another life experience that identifies you as a living, breathing, healthy woman.

To give you a preview of what to expect, this woman's description of menopause probably represents the mainstream and may help you understand what it is all about.

Menopause was quite an experience for me. My periods got a little crazy, then became shorter and shorter, and finally stopped. My hot flashes started before then but didn't reach their crescendo until later. And for the better part of a year, I had bad PMS and felt terribly fragile. There were other major events happening in my life at the time, so I can't attribute all of my emotional outbursts to hormonal change, but I know it played a major role. I'd be standing in the supermarket and just start to cry without any warning whatsoever. Clearly, menopause was a time for me when forces other than outside influences ruled my body and mind.

Married mother, 52

What Is Menopause?

Menopause is the cessation of menstruation, usually defined as one year after your last period. No more. No less.

Yet common usage of the word *menopause* often means many other experiences, such as the beginning of menopausal signs, the years following your last menstrual period, or an entire phase of your life. Phrases like "going through menopause" and "just starting menopause" are common.

To be more precise, the following terms will be used throughout this book:

Perimenopause. This refers to the transition between when you first start to experience menopausal signs, typically in your 40s, until the time your period stops, usually around the age of 51. During this time, most women experience changes in their menstrual patterns and some may have hot flashes and mood swings. Perimenopause usually lasts for an average of six years, although it can be as short as one year or go on for ten years.

It's crazy living with a woman in her 40s. It used to be that you could count on a couple of bad days a month. Now, my wife has PMS, menopause, perimenopause, and everything else. I kid her that I get about a week a month window of opportunity when she's actually normal!

Married father, 44

Postmenopause. Obviously, this is the time after you pass menopause. In other words, it begins approximately one year after your last period and continues for the rest of your life. The most common signs of menopause such as hot flashes, vaginal dryness, and mood swings tend to appear toward the end of perimenopause and may extend into postmenopause.

Climacteric. Completely unrelated to any form of sexual arousal, this word describes the entire rite of passage beginning with perimenopause and including postmenopause. *Climacteric* is a term used primarily by the medical community to refer succinctly to the complete menopause time span and the accompanying endocrine, somatic (body), and psychic changes. Instead of the more technical term *climacteric, menopause* will be used in the following pages to describe this entire rite of passage.

When Will It Happen and How Long Will It Last?

One of the most difficult aspects of life is unpredictability. The good news is that women tend to have menopause around the same age. Most women are 51 when they experience menopause, and that age has remained constant in recorded history. Ironically, because the average life expectancy for a woman in 1900 was only 48 years old, it has not been until recently that large numbers of women lived long enough to experience menopause. Today, women live well into their 70s and 80s and, with knowledge about midlife issues, have the opportunity to make their postmenopausal years as healthy as possible.

The less wonderful news is about the wide age range for women starting perimenopause. Some begin in their early 40s, others in their mid- or late 40s. Although it is comforting to know that you will most likely start perimenopause sometime in your fifth decade, ten years is a large time span to consider.

The truth of the matter is that many women avoid thinking

about it completely and greet changes in their bodies with denial. I remember chatting with a friend a year older than I after I had just started to experience signs of perimenopause—a couple of hot flashes and very irregular periods. I mentioned that I was starting to go through menopause and she responded with horror, disbelief, and concern. Horror that I could even think that I was old enough to be menopausal, disbelief that it was happening to a friend her own age, and concern that I see a doctor right away because my diagnosis was incorrect and I was undoubtedly suffering from some dread disease.

Several years later and after reading many magazine and newspaper articles on menopause, my friend has come around to some degree, although she still clings to the idea that nothing will really happen to her until she is 49 or 50. She may be right, but it is best to prepare yourself for the changes that come with perimenopause so that you are not caught off guard.

Unfortunately, there is no correlation between when you first start to menstruate and when you reach menopause. With that in mind, take a look at the table below to see how the average age range actually breaks down. Note that only 5 percent of women continue to menstruate after 55.

AGE OF WOMEN	PERCENTAGE PAST MENOPAUSE
47	25
50	50
52	75
55	95

Source: Robin Marantz Henig, *How a Woman Ages* (New York: Ballantine Books, 1985), p. 111. Taken from the Diagram Group, *Woman's Body: An Owner's Manual* (London: Paddington Press, 1977), p. F-02.

To figure out where you might fit in this chart, read through the following list of variables.

- *If your mother* started perimenopause in her mid-40s, you probably will too. Genetics is a significant determining factor and unless you fit some of the following descriptions, you should expect to reach menopause about the same time your mother did. However, while the approximate time frame may be similar between mother and daughter, the nature of the menopausal experience may be different. There is no reason to panic if your mother had a difficult menopause—research indicates a hereditary relationship for the onset of menopause but does not show a correlation between mother and daughter menopausal signs. This is a good time to cast away the kind of anxiety about menopause that this woman has because of her mother's experience.

My greatest fear about menopause is that I'll repeat the emotional imbalance my mother went through. She screamed for five years and was totally out of control. Maybe it was because she was a first-grade teacher and had to curb her temper in school. But believe me, when she got home, we all took it on the chin.

Single mother, 51

- *If your mother had poor nutrition during her pregnancy with you,* you will probably have an earlier menopause.
- *If your menstrual cycles were shorter than average,* there is a good chance you will experience menopause two years earlier than women with longer cycles. In a recent study, researchers found that women between 20 and 35 who had menstrual cycles of less than twenty-six days reached menopause earlier than women with cycles of thirty-three days or more.
- *If you delivered five or more children,* it is likely that you will experience menopause one year later than women who have not had any children. Each delivery seems to delay the onset of menopause by a few months, so the more children you've had, the later you will reach menopause.
- *If you had your first child after 40,* you are more likely to have a later than average menopause.
- *If you smoke more than fifteen cigarettes a day,* you will reach menopause two to three years earlier than nonsmokers.

However, if you quit, you will probably be able to cut the time down to one year.

- *If you are thin and small boned,* you will most likely have an earlier menopause than average.
- *If you are heavy and short,* you will probably have a later menopause than most women.
- *If you used birth control pills consistently for many years,* you may experience a slightly later onset of menopause.
- *If you had a hysterectomy or tubal ligation* many years before the average age of menopause, you will probably reach menopause earlier than you would have naturally. This holds true whether or not you still have your ovaries.
- *If you are left-handed,* there is a chance you will experience menopause three to five years earlier than right-handed women. Based on a recent study of Mexican-American women, researchers theorize this is a result of more frequent autoimmune disorders in left-handers, which may affect hormonal levels and trigger earlier menopause.

Now that you have some information to work with, you can calculate when you might start perimenopause or experience menopause. Clearly, this is not a precise exercise, but it will give you a framework for what you can expect and when. This is how the exercise worked out for me.

First I assumed I would have a full six years of perimenopause and noted that my mother reached menopause at 49. I then reviewed the variables and discovered I had an earlier menopause profile:

- A short menstrual cycle of twenty-six days.
- A thin body on a very small-boned frame.
- Not bearing children.

Working backward from my mother's menopause age of 49, I found it was logical that I started perimenopause on the early side at 42, which is exactly what happened—irregular periods, more intense premenstrual syndrome (PMS) mood swings, and even a couple of hot flashes. This meant I would probably reach menopause sooner than my mother, when I reach 48 or earlier if my perimenopause did not continue for the full six-year average. As I am 46 and still perimenopausal, the jury is out on the final outcome.

Becoming menopausal is not a competitive sport. There is no real upside to having it earlier than later, nor is there any benefit to having a more intense experience. Although it is a universal phenomenon, all women go through it differently sooner or later. This woman in her early 40s expresses some of the confusion around menopause and the anxiety that goes along with not knowing what is going to happen to you.

When I'm with my friends and I think about menopause, I have the same reaction I did when we all got our periods . . . Who's going to get it first? Who's going to blaze the trail? In some ways there would be the same somebody-got-there-first feeling. But I'm so glad it isn't me . . . this must mean that I'm younger. There are all those issues that aren't talked about—the competitive feelings of when people turn 40 first, before you. Whew! But in some ways, those people are the pioneers . . . they're experiencing something you're not and in a way, you're left out.

Married woman, 41

False Promises

Now that you have an understanding of what facts you can count on, it is time to dispel some long-standing menopausal myths.

False: The more menstrual problems you have—PMS, cramps—the more problems you will have with menopause. There is no scientific evidence linking severe menopause signs with problematic menstrual cycles. For some women, the opposite is true, with menstrual patterns improving during perimenopause.

False: The age you first started menstruating determines the age of menopause. If only this were true, you could easily predict the onset of perimenopause. Again, the most influential factor in determining when you will experience menopause is your mother's history.

False: Menopause causes depression and mental illness. Perhaps the most famous and enduring myth, it has proven false in several recent scientific studies. A landmark research project involving 2,500 women 45 to 55 years old concluded that middle-aged women were no more likely to be depressed than other women. What's more, according to a 1990 clinical study, for the vast majority of healthy middle-aged women, menopause does not lead to emotional instability or psychological problems. However, sleep deprivation brought on by midlife hormonal shifts can often make it harder to cope with normal day-to-day stress. Consequently, employment problems, marriage difficulties, financial insecurity, and issues with children and aging parents can have a stronger negative influence on a woman's mental health. During perimenopause, hormonal swings can also increase the likelihood of premenstrual mood changes.

Signs of Menopause

With good reason, menopause is often compared to puberty as another rite of passage in a woman's life. Take a few minutes and think back to the beginning of your teenage years and the first signs of your body changing—growing breasts, pimples, pubic hair. It was scary, exciting, obvious, irreversible, and out of your control. Now remember how you felt when you got your first period—a little strange, relieved, and perhaps self-conscious. There was no longer any doubt you were becoming a woman.

Menopause occurs in the same measured way. Gradually and, in most cases, naturally, your body changes to prepare for the next phase of life. It does not happen overnight with monthly periods coming to a screeching halt. Instead there are real physical markers, just as in your teenage years, that indicate the beginning of perimenopause. The first signs are quite obvious if you know what to look for.

One woman, who had her last child in her late 30s, gained some perspective on her own menopausal transition as she watched her daughter enter puberty.

> It's interesting to watch the changes in my body as they compare to what my teenage daughter is experiencing. Her straight figure is becoming curvaceous at the same time that my curves are starting to straighten out. Just before my period each month, I seem to thicken through the center. I find it fascinating that it's beyond my control.
>
> Somehow, I don't have as clear a picture of menopause as I did of puberty. I knew much more about what was happening when I was a teenager. I knew the facts of life and all my friends had their periods before me. So I not only knew about it, but I had seen it and sort of experienced it vicariously.
>
> This time, I've only had a couple of friends who talked to me about menopause. Yet I have more insight into what is happening with my body now than I did when I was 13 or 14.
>
> Married mother, 50

Changing Menstrual Patterns

Most women first notice small changes in their monthly periods. Some time during your 40s, your periods may become slightly heavier or lighter, last longer or only a couple of days, or alter the cycle time—twenty-six days instead of the usual thirty, thirty-four days instead of twenty-eight. Whatever your situation, the most important thing to recognize is a difference in your normal menstrual experience.

What's more, your "new" menstrual pattern will continue to change as you approach menopause. There is no standard or typical perimenopausal menstrual cycle. Just to give you an idea of the wide range of possibilities, 324 women who were followed for three years in a recent study of menstrual cycle lengths reported eighty-one different patterns.

Remember, menopause is defined as being one year after your last period. Scientists found that if you are between 45 and 49 years old and have not menstruated for seven months, there is less than a 50 percent chance you have actually reached menopause.

PMS

You probably know quite a bit about PMS, but you might not be aware that it is often an early indicator of perimenopause. Many doctors believe that PMS can start or intensify in your late 30s and continue through perimenopause. The familiar signs can include monthly breast tenderness, bloating, weight gain, depression, anxiety, irritability, and insomnia.

I usually am very up and I have an even disposition. I realized I would wake up at times and just not feel happy. There wasn't anything going on in my life that would make me unhappy. In fact, everything was wonderful. But for some reason I was just oversensitive. I can remember being in the kitchen one night fixing a gourmet dinner for my husband. I just love to cook and I go all out. I did a four-course dinner and really had fun. Later that evening I went to clean the stove and he said, "Honey, I'll clean it for you." "Oh, I can clean the stove by myself," I said. "Listen, you've been in the kitchen all day making dinner. The least I can do is help you with the dishes. I'll take care of the stove and the pots and pans, and if you want to load the dishwasher, I'll give you a hand," he said. I answered angrily, "Do you think I'm not capable of cleaning my own kitchen?"

All of a sudden, I stopped myself, and my husband just looked at me and said, "What's wrong?" I said I didn't know.

That was the first sign. It was the first time that it ever really dawned on me that I was saying things I'd never said before. Now we joke about it. Whenever my husband says, "I'll clean the stove for you," I look him straight in the eye and say, "Don't you think I can clean the stove just as well as you can?" and we laugh.

Married woman, 45

Sleep Changes

Recent neuroendocrine research done at Yale University indicates that women experience restless, fragmented sleep five to seven years before menopause. Sleep changes are often the earliest indicators of hormonal change.

Hot Flashes

An amazing and still perplexing phenomenon, hot flashes are experienced by 85 percent of all women. Although you are not alone in this experience, the first one is always a surprise. It usually starts like a deep blush, with heat emanating from your upper chest into your neck, face, and arms. Your skin actually reddens, your pulse speeds up, and you break out in a sweat. Fortunately, it only lasts a few minutes, but for some it can occur frequently and be quite uncomfortable (see Chapter 2, "What's Going to Happen to Me? . . . Perimenopause").

This woman's experience with hot flashes is not uncommon.

I think the worst thing about menopause is the hot flashes. If during the day I can get through with maybe two flashes instead of ten, I figure I'm way ahead. I'll just be sitting around completely dressed and then all of a sudden I feel as if I'm a chicken in a rotisserie.

When I get a flash now, I can deal with it because I know how. I don't have a problem with it anymore. I used to think people were looking at me. But I don't get red; I just get terribly hot and uncomfortable. It's just a part of my life right now. It's like . . . so what?

Single mother, 59

Vaginal Dryness

Seldom discussed among women and rarely mentioned to a mate, vaginal dryness plagues many women and is common during the latter phase of perimenopause. As estrogen production diminishes, the vaginal area becomes less moist. During intercourse, lubrication takes longer, and unless properly stimulated, some women will experience painful sex. This is not the end of your

sex life, for vaginal dryness can be quickly and effectively reversed. It is just a matter of understanding what is happening to
your body and then making a decision to do something about it
(see Chapter 2, "What's Going to Happen to Me? . . . Perimenopause" and Chapter 7, "Sex").

Urinary Stress Incontinence

This is an uncomfortable and embarrassing occurrence that happens to many women at one time or another during perimenopause and menopause. Under certain conditions, you may
momentarily lose control of your bladder, releasing a very small
amount of urine. It is most likely to occur in physical stress
situations like jogging, aerobics, laughing, or coughing.

Do not panic. This is not a permanent condition, but simply
a result of weakened pelvic and bladder muscles due to changing
estrogen levels in your body. Like any weak muscles, specific
exercise can strengthen and bring them back to normal (see
Chapter 2, "What's Going to Happen to Me? . . . Perimenopause").

Diagnostic Tests

With what you now understand about the signs of menopause
and when they might occur, you probably feel more comfortable
about what is happening to your body. However, many women
still want to know exactly where they stand: How low is my
estrogen level? Am I at risk for heart disease and osteoporosis? Is
my irregular bleeding all because of menopause? This is the right
time to see a doctor and get a more professional opinion.

Because of all the changes happening in your body as you
approach menopause, it is important to make sure they are part
of the natural process and not indicators that something else
might be wrong. During this time period and into postmenopause, your physician will probably give you tests you have never
had before.

There are many diagnostic tests available and just as many

reasons for employing them. Some of them will be new to you, and others, although familiar, may be used differently. Therefore, it is helpful to understand what a specific test measures, why it is important, and what can be done with the results.

Listed below are tests most often ordered for women in the menopausal years.

Test	**Dual Photon (DPA) and Dual X-Ray (DEXA) Absorptiometry**
Measurement	Bone density (bone mineral content).
Indication	Perimenopause, family history of osteoporosis, thin body, use of thyroid medication or steroids, heavy alcohol intake.
Procedure	These tests measure bone mineral content anywhere in the body. Painless.
Results	Your risk for osteoporosis will be determined based on the level of your bone mineral content. The results will also be used as a baseline to monitor your bone mineral content from year to year.
Test	**Follicle-Stimulating Hormone (FSH)**
Measurement	Estrogen level.
Indication	Changing menstrual pattern, hot flashes, urinary incontinence.
Procedure	A blood test is taken each month for at least two successive months. Blood should be drawn on the first or second day of monthly bleeding for the most accurate results.
Results	Women with FSH levels at or above 8 international units are probably six years or less from menopause. If FSH

levels are high and exceed 30 international units, your body is not producing significant estrogen. Menopause is usually diagnosed at this time if periods have also stopped.

Test	**Endometrial or Intrauterine Biopsy**
Measurement	Endometrial cancer or hyperplasia.
Indication	Heavy or irregular vaginal bleeding.
Procedure	Tissue from the endometrial lining is collected using suction with either a narrow tube or a hollow cutting instrument attached to a syringe. The procedure is usually performed in a doctor's office and lasts two to three minutes. Mildly uncomfortable to severe cramping.
Results	There is a 95 percent accuracy rate in detection of cancer and hyperplasia. Depending on the diagnosis, a D&C (dilatation and curettage) may be necessary as a follow-up.

Test	**Lipid Profile**
Measurement	Cholesterol and triglyceride blood levels.
Indication	Routine annual physical, perimenopause, overweight, family history of heart disease.
Procedure	A blood test is taken after a twelve- to fourteen-hour fast.
Results	Accurate measurements of your high-density lipoproteins, low-density lipoproteins, and triglycerides will help determine your risk for heart disease.

Test	**Mammogram**
Measurement	Screening for breast growths and cancer.
Indication	Routine annual physical after age 40, perimenopause, family history of breast cancer.
Procedure	The breasts are examined by mechanically flattening them with a machine and taking an X ray. The procedure lasts four to five seconds for each breast. Mildly uncomfortable.
Results	Unless a specific growth is discovered, the results will be used as a baseline to monitor change in your breasts from year to year.

Test	**Ovarian Hormone Profile**
Measurement	Levels of estradiol (the primary human estrogen), testosterone, and progesterone.
Indication	Changing sleep patterns, worsening PMS symptoms, irregular menses, hot flashes, loss of libido, vaginal changes.
Procedure	Blood samples are taken on day 1 (first day of monthly bleeding) and day 20 of the menstrual cycle to determine a declining baseline production of these hormones as well as any significant rate of change throughout the menstrual cycle.
Results	Blood levels of estradiol less than 50 picograms per milliliter are associated with increased frequency of hot flashes, sleep changes, and sexual difficulties. Testosterone levels less than 30 nanograms per milliliter are associ-

ated with diminished sex drive. Progesterone levels greater than 5 milligrams per milliliter on day 20 indicate ovulation is still occurring and pregnancy is possible.

Test	**Pap Test**
Measurement	Malignant and premalignant condition of the vagina, cervix, and endometrium.
Indication	Routine annual physical, unexplained vaginal bleeding.
Procedure	A swab is taken from the vaginal walls and uterine lining. Painless.
Results	If a malignant or premalignant condition is discovered, other tests may be prescribed to confirm the diagnosis.

Test	**Progesterone Challenge**
Measurement	Screening for endometrial cancer or hyperplasia.
Indication	Irregular periods during perimenopause, heavy or breakthrough vaginal bleeding.
Procedure	The doctor will prescribe 10 milligrams of progestin a day for seven days.
Results	If periods become regular in flow and timing, you are probably all right; otherwise an endometrial biopsy may be requested to develop a diagnosis.

Test	**Vaginal Smear**
Measurement	Estrogen level.
Indication	Changing menstrual pattern, hot flashes, urinary incontinence.

Procedure	A swab is taken from the inner third of the lateral vaginal wall. It is administered as part of a routine pelvic exam. Painless.
Results	If a low estrogen profile is discovered, other tests may be prescribed to confirm the diagnosis of menopause. Results from vaginal smear testing are not as reliable as blood level testing such as an ovarian hormone profile.
Test	**Vaginal Sonography**
Measurement	The thickness of the uterine lining, existing cysts, endometrial hyperplasia and ovarian cancer.
Indication	Routine annual physical (in the future), unexplained vaginal bleeding, changing menstrual pattern.
Procedure	A thin plastic ultrasound probe is inserted inside the vagina and swept along the uterine walls. It allows the physician to clearly view the ovaries and uterus. Painless.
Results	This is an excellent measurement of the endometrium. Depending on thickness (5 millimeters or greater), an endometrial biopsy may be required.

Keep in mind this is only a partial list of tests your doctor may order during your menopausal years. Think of this list as a guide to help you ask the right questions at the right time. Obviously, severe problems may require different measurement and analysis.

Adjusting to Change

Menopause may not be the end of the world, but it is the finale of certain familiar bodily functions. It is this ending that can cause sadness about what no longer exists and anxiety about the future. As a woman, you have already been through a myriad of significant bodily changes, some of which were no fun at all, but you survived, as you will again after menopause.

> *I really have a problem with menopause because it marks the beginning of the downhill slide toward old age. Everything I've read talks about how a woman's body changes after menopause and I don't like it one little bit. And if I had a way to reverse it, to keep my periods forever, I'd do it in a flash. Bleeding once a month never bothered me and not having my period anymore is like saying my youth has ended.*
>
> Married mother, 47

This is a big change for your body and it represents a watershed transition for all women. The issue is how you decide to deal with it. Yes, you do have a choice, even if you are part of the 25 percent of women who have intense hot flashes and other menopausal indicators. Not knowing exactly what will happen to you during menopause and how you will emerge after it is over is probably the greatest source of fear and anxiety. Most women's mothers never did talk to them about menopause, and what women have gleaned from rumor, brief magazine articles, and media sound bites has done little to fill that knowledge gap. By reading this book, you are already way ahead of the game—knowledge is power. So, too, is your desire to take action and feel more in control. This is the kind of behavior that will make the menopausal transition easier.

However, for some women, menopause can be a convenient event that allows them to hide out. They use menopause as a raison d'être to avoid other issues looming in the wings. It could even be called the "brass ring of excuses." After all, only you know how you feel, and you may be able to use your brass ring for five to ten years or longer.

As you enter your middle years, menopause is just one of many changes that lie ahead. Your 40s and 50s are decades during which your parents may become ill or even die, children become adolescent or leave home, and careers—both yours and that of your partner—may shift dramatically. It is also a time when you can finally sit back a little and enjoy some of your accomplishments. You no longer feel the need to become queen of the universe and you have a much clearer picture of who you are and what you want to do with your life, all of which will help you cope with change.

This woman has a refreshing attitude about change and the aging process that you may find helpful.

> *Menopause is really the first time I thought about getting old. But the key to aging well, or maybe not aging much at all, is being open to new experiences. I mean open to new ideas and new ways of dealing with things . . . like menopause. It was easy to be flexible in your 20s and 30s, but we seemed to get set in our ways by the time we reached 40. I just think getting older is a whole new ball game if you can free up your thinking, maybe throw out previous ways of operating, and look at everything with a new perspective.*
> *Single woman, 49*

Midlife and menopause are a challenge but one you can get through more easily by maintaining a positive attitude and an understanding that this, too, will pass.

Chapter Two

What's Going to Happen to Me? . . . Perimenopause

*I know all about your woman's troubles there, Edith, but
when I had the hernia that time, I didn't make you wear
the truss. No, no, no, Edith . . . if you're going to have
a change of life, you gotta do it right now. I'm going to
give you just 30 seconds. That's it!*
    —Archie Bunker, "Edith's Problem,"
        All in the Family

So here you are in your 40s, with your life somewhat under
control. You know who you are, pretty much where you are
headed, and how you are going to get there. During the past
twenty years, you have also gotten to know your body—what you
can expect it to do, when it will get tired, how it functions each
month, its ups and downs.

Then along comes perimenopause. Slowly and inconspicu-
ously. You probably would not even notice unless you took some
time to know the signs and what to look for: periods a little off
schedule; perhaps more intense mood swings than usual; sore
breasts all month long; sweating at night, disrupting your sleep.

What is going on here?

This is perimenopause, the beginning of menopause. Perimenopause is a transition period between when you first start to
experience menopausal signs, usually in your 40s, until the time
your period stops, typically around the age of 51.

Yes, this is really happening to you. No, you are not too
young. And yes, you will get through this period of your life the

same way you made it through adolescence. You will learn a lot more about your body than you ever expected. You will also end up with a greater feeling of comfort and familiarity with yourself as a woman.

> *It may sound crazy, but I'm kind of excited about starting meno-pause. I feel it's sort of interesting to be going through this— interesting in the way that pregnancy is interesting—that your body is going to do all these new things. I always wonder why men don't try growing a beard at least once. How could you resist seeing what you'd look like? There is that kind of adventure in it. And there's the excitement of moving on to a new stage. Almost like graduation—there is no turning back.*
>
> Married mother, 50

Anatomy 101—Relearning the Basics

In order to understand what happens to your body during peri-menopause, you need to review the nuts and bolts of menstrua-tion. This is not a simple assignment. Most of us first learned about menstruation from our mothers, with the details filled in by books, friends, or teachers' explanations. Knowledge from sources like these will not help very much at this point.

The menstrual cycle is complex and affects many different parts of your body. It is essential to figure out how it all works. With this understanding, you will be in a strong position to decide how you want to handle your menopause, and it will help you make clear choices about hormone replacement therapy and alternative treatment.

The Short Version

Once your body is capable of reproduction, it prepares itself each month for conception by releasing specific amounts of various hormones, including estrogen, to control the process. The men-strual cycle lasts an average of twenty-eight days and is orches-trated by hormones. During the first half of the cycle, known as the *follicular phase*, which lasts ten to seventeen days, these hormones act on your body to

- Develop, protect, and nourish an egg.
- Create follicles (sacs that hold the eggs) in the ovary.
- Thicken the walls of the uterus by increasing the blood supply.
- Push a single follicle toward the surface of the ovary.

About halfway through the cycle, the follicle that has been pushing against the wall of the ovary ruptures, releasing an egg in a process called *ovulation*.

Meanwhile the ruptured follicle will begin to produce other hormones, including progesterone, for the second half, or *luteal phase*, of the cycle, lasting thirteen to fifteen days, to

- Further develop the thickened walls of the uterus in preparation for pregnancy.
- Prevent the growth of any more follicles to start a new cycle.

If pregnancy does not occur, hormone levels decrease, the thickened lining of the womb is shed in menstruation, and a signal is eventually sent to start a new cycle.

The Details

Each of the two phases of the menstrual cycle is governed by its own set of hormones, and the secretion of one impacts on the other. There are several other hormones in addition to estrogen and progesterone, briefly described here, and they each have a specific and complex role in the reproductive cycle.

- *Gonadotropin-releasing hormone* (GRH) stimulates the pituitary gland to release follicle-stimulating hormone (FSH).
- *FSH* stimulates development of follicles in the ovary.
- *Estrogen* stimulates growth of the uterine lining.

- *Luteinizing hormone* (LH) causes ovulation and transforms the ruptured follicle into the corpus luteum, which then produces progesterone.
- *Progesterone* makes the lining of the uterus more receptive to the egg; prepares the body for pregnancy by increasing your appetite, metabolic rate, and fluid retention; increases secretion of the oil glands, often causing oily hair and acne; and prevents the pituitary gland from releasing FSH and LH, thus halting the growth of more follicles.

In addition to biological changes, these hormones can also activate subtle emotional changes during your cycle. For example, during the first half of the cycle, women usually feel emotionally relaxed yet alert and self-confident, with a sense of well-being. As ovulation occurs, they often become highly responsive and assertive. Then during the second phase, women may experience a series of negatively toned emotions like heightened arousal, tension, and anxiety. Try to keep track of how you are feeling during one or two of your menstrual cycles to see if your emotions follow these patterns.

Why bother knowing all these details? Because during perimenopause, your normal cycle will begin to change and possibly affect your body in a variety of ways. If you have a firm grasp of how everything works before menopause, it makes it easier to identify the changes as they happen during perimenopause. You will feel less confused and anxious about this natural transition. However, you may still have strong emotional feelings about this irrevocable change, as expressed by this woman on the cusp of perimenopause.

I'm 44 and I'm not really seeing very many signs. I expect I probably will within the next six or seven years. But when I think about menopause, I think about finality. The finality that takes place when the whole reproductive system goes through its last course of changes. You don't have choices anymore and it feels like an ending. There is no question that my body is changing already.

I notice more wrinkles and gray hair, and my stamina is not what it used to be. Not that it's disappeared, but it's a totally different picture from the way it was in my early 30s and light-years away from my 20s. As I look back on those earlier phases, I can see the aging process with more clarity than I ever have before.

I don't feel good about having less vitality and strength. And I don't feel good about the other changes in my face and body. There are certain things we can do to prolong youth, to pamper the skin that wrinkles and color the hair that grays. But there's not really anything we can do about the aging process. I guess I feel accepting, but there's not much of a choice. And no longer having a choice is still a loss in my mind.

Married woman, 44

Swan Song of the Ovaries

With more detailed knowledge of the menstrual cycle, you can see the pivotal role the ovaries and the eggs they contain play in the action of hormones in your body. It is like a ballet, carefully choreographed with a stunning beginning, exciting midpart, and an inevitable but gradual finale.

You start out at about twenty weeks, still in your mother's uterus, with all the eggs you will ever have—an astounding total of about 10 million. From that point, you begin to lose them on a monthly basis, similar to a menstrual cycle, until at birth you have around 2 million eggs left. This process of monthly egg reduction continues throughout childhood, adolescence, and adulthood until, by the time you reach your 40s, some of the remaining eggs just do not function like they used to. They may not respond to various hormones, or if they do and stimulate the production of estrogen and progesterone, it may not be in exactly the right combination or the timing may be off.

This obviously raises havoc with your body and can give you some or all of the signs of perimenopause.

By the time you are 51, the few eggs you may have left will not function properly, your ovaries will stop producing estrogen and progesterone in any significant amount, and you will stop menstruating.

Decreasing Ovarian Function and How It Affects Your Body

You have seen how hormones working in tandem control the menstrual cycle. However, once your ovaries start to produce less estrogen and progesterone, as they do in your 40s, the hormonal balance is thrown off and your entire reproductive system is affected:

- With fewer eggs in the ovaries, the number of follicles to hold them is reduced.
- Fewer follicles means a decrease in fertility.
- Altered hormone production results in abnormal menstrual cycles and faulty signals sent to other hormone activators.
- Even though it gets faulty signals or no signal at all, the pituitary continues to release FSH and LH in the hope of stimulating the ovary.
- Closer to menopause, follicles no longer mature completely and estrogen production decreases.
- Ovulation stops occurring, thus no progesterone is produced at all.
- Without progesterone to counteract it, the uterine lining continues to thicken and eventually is shed in bits and pieces rather than a single, normal menstrual flow.

These significant hormonal changes will also cause very specific effects during perimenopause. As mentioned in Chapter 1, you will probably experience irregular menstrual bleeding and may be disturbed by hot flashes, vaginal dryness, incontinence, and mood swings.

Caught unaware, this perimenopausal woman suffered needlessly until she figured out what was happening to her body.

My period started to become very irregular. I was one of those people who used to get it every twenty-eight days on the dot, but in my late 30s, it started getting weird. At the same time I gradually became dryer and dryer and sex turned into a very painful event. I didn't know what was going on, which is striking to me in retrospect. I'm pretty knowledgeable, fairly bright, do a lot of reading, and know about my body. But it never occurred to me what was going on. I just thought I was having some strange psychological resistance to sex. Maybe we weren't having enough foreplay or I was telling myself I wasn't attracted to my husband anymore. I didn't understand that there was a logical and real reason behind all of it. Now that I know, it's a psychological blessing to me to realize that I'm not crazy and that there are ways to deal with the dryness, like lubricating myself. I'm shopping around for a lubricant I like and already feel much better about the whole situation.

Married woman, 43

Fortunately, decreased ovarian function does not happen all at once, except in the case of surgical menopause (hysterectomy) or chemically induced menopause (chemotherapy) (see Chapter 8, "Special Problems"). Your ovaries do not just shrivel and die. In fact, they continue to produce hormones in gradually lessening amounts right up until menopause. Even in the first few years of postmenopause, your ovaries will continue to produce very small amounts of estrogen beneficial to your body.

Menstrual Bleeding . . . The Ebb and Flow

Change in your normal menstrual bleeding pattern is usually the first sign of perimenopause. Some women experience lighter or heavier bleeding while others discover their monthly cycle changing in the number of days. If you pay close attention, you may be able to distinguish some changes as early as your late 30s. However, every woman is different.

A small number of lucky women, roughly 10 to 15 percent, wake up one month and never have another period again; they have regular monthly periods until sometime in their 40s and then just stop. This does not happen very often.

There is also a small group of women who bleed almost continually throughout perimenopause right up until the end—a terrible prospect, but no one has ever bled to death from perimenopause.

More commonly, women start having irregular, unpredictable periods—sometimes heavy, sometimes light—but generally diminishing in flow over time.

Behind the Scenes

Think of this time in your life in a linear fashion with regular twenty-eight-day menstrual cycles on one end and menopause with no monthly bleeding on the other end. In the middle is perimenopause, an extended time of unpredictable menstrual behavior. At any given time during perimenopause, you can be closer to one end than to the other. Examples are given in the following table.

INDICATOR	SCENARIO
If your cycles are shorter . . .	Preovulatory estrogen is not being made as well, and the follicular phase of your cycle shrinks from the usual fourteen days. You still ovulate and still have your period two weeks later, but your cycle is shorter.
If your breasts are sore throughout your cycle . . .	You are probably not ovulating and thus not producing progesterone. This results in an effect similar to pregnancy, when estrogen is produced and not opposed by progesterone.
If your monthly bleeding is light . . .	You are producing less estrogen than usual. Thus, your uterine lining will be thinner and less

| If your monthly bleeding is heavy . . . | flow will occur during menstruation. |
| | You are probably not ovulating and estrogen continues to stimulate the growth of the uterine lining with no progesterone to stop it. It will grow until estrogen production finally stops and the lining, which is now much heavier than usual, is shed. |

These possible behind-the-scenes descriptions give you an idea of the effect of the hormonal changes on the rest of your body. However, they are not meant to be used as self-diagnostic tools, and you should discuss changes in your menstrual pattern with your doctor on an ongoing basis. More important, any breakthrough or unexplained vaginal bleeding is a signal that something abnormal could be going on. It is essential that you respond quickly and see a physician about it right away.

Staying in Control

One of the most frustrating aspects of perimenopause is not knowing exactly when you might have menstrual bleeding. With a changing menstrual pattern, it is almost impossible to remember what happened month to month and you can easily lose track of when to expect your period. All of a sudden you start bleeding, perhaps have an embarrassing accident, and feel like you are going through adolescence all over again.

> I like to be in control; that's why menopause scares me. I get paralyzed by the thought that something could happen that I won't be able to control and it will affect my life, whether it's my performance at work or my ability to be a wife or a mother or whatever. I feel very insecure about that prospect.
>
> Married mother, 47

There are a few things you can do to feel more in control of the situation. First of all, as the Boy Scout motto cautions, be prepared. Do not go out without some sort of sanitary protection. Ever. In the same way you remember to carry your keys, be sure to bring along a tampon or pad all the time. With their trim, neat packaging, they can easily be slipped into a coat pocket, briefcase, or purse. Do not let yourself get caught. Think of it as a game and enjoy the sweet victory of outwitting your changing body.

The second thing you can do is keep an ongoing chart of your changing cycle. Tedious as this may seem, it will give you a point of reference each month and will be quite helpful in discussing your perimenopausal signs with a doctor. The key to maintaining an ongoing chart or log is to do it in a way that is easiest for you. Some people fill in an existing calendar, others keep a running list of dates and events. Whatever works for you is fine. Just be sure to record the following in some way or another.

1. Regular monthly bleeding.
   - Note beginning and end: morning, afternoon, or evening.
   - Specify type of flow: normal, heavy, or light.
   - Indicate other symptoms if appropriate: cramps, breast soreness, bloating, or moodiness.
2. Breakthrough bleeding (bleeding or staining occurring at times other than the end of your monthly cycle).
   - Note beginning and end.
   - Specify type of flow: normal, heavy, or light.
   - Note color: dark or normal.
     Remember, breakthrough bleeding is often an indication of abnormality and should be investigated right away by your physician. Take it seriously.
3. Ovulation if possible (some women feel a short, mild cramp around the middle of their cycle).
   - Note date.

If you keep a record faithfully, you will have a more accurate picture of what is actually happening each month as opposed to relying on your memory for answers. You will also be in a better position to outguess your body and predict what will happen next. Below is a sample chart to get you started.

Menstrual Cycle Chart

	START DATE	END DATE	TYPE OF FLOW	NUMBER OF TAMPONS	NOTES	DUR- ATION (DAYS)	DAYS SINCE LAST PERIOD
Regular period	3/10	3/15	Heavy	20	Sore breasts, cramps	6	25
Regular period	4/9	4/12	Light	12	Cranky, anxious	4	30
Break- through bleeding	4/21	4/22	Light	5	Cramps	2	9
Regular period	5/6	5/9	Moderate	15	Snappish for 1 day	4	27

The third option, especially if you are plagued by heavy irregular bleeding, is to discuss progesterone therapy with your doctor. Progestin, taken in doses of 10 milligrams for seven consecutive days, will cause your uterine lining to shed predictably every month. It is also an excellent way to ensure you have no excessive buildup of your endometrium. Eventually, when you stop making sufficient amounts of estrogen, your periods will stop even if you continue to take progestin. However, many women do not respond well to this hormone, and you may have to experiment with different brands to find one that works for you (see Chapter 4, "Hormone Replacement Therapy").

Hot Flashes

Resign yourself. Eighty-five percent of all women experience hot flashes and still live to tell the tale. Hot flashes are not the end of the world, but are startling, strange, unpredictable, uncomfortable, unexplained, and, except when bobsledding in Alaska, unwelcome.

> *What bothered me the most was hot flashes. During the day, it was embarrassing because other people were not warm and I was hot. I conduct seminars and remember being in front of a room, praying, "Please don't have a hot flash, not now." I kept turning away from the group to wipe my face. The flashes seemed to happen at random times. I could be sitting in a restaurant and suddenly become drenched in sweat or riding in a car continually opening and closing windows because one minute I'm cold and the next minute I'm hot. I managed to cope during the day, but nighttime was the big problem. I was up all night either with hot flashes or just plain old insomnia. I was a zombie and in tears most of the time from lack of sleep. I couldn't stand anything touching my body—a sheet, a nightgown, pajamas, anything. And I would wake up in the morning absolutely knocked out as if I'd been up all night in a prizefight.*
>
> Single woman, 53

The phenomenon of hot flashes still remains a mystery to modern medicine with many questions left unanswered. What causes hot flashes? Why do some women escape them? Why are flashes more frequent and severe for some? Why do certain women have them for years but others only experience them briefly?

According to Dr. Fredi Kronenberg, professor of physiology at Columbia University, "Hot flashes have been known for a long time and are recognized as being associated with menopause. They've been treated with various ovary extracts for over one hundred years—we didn't have pure estrogen way back then; they were grinding up ovaries and giving it to women—yet we don't know why estrogen relieves hot flashes. It's pretty amazing that after all this time we still don't have the answers. But it has only been within the past fifteen years that people have seriously studied the physiology of hot flashes."

Neuroendocrine research done by Dr. Phillip Sarrel of Yale University's departments of obstetrics and gynecology and psychiatry and by others at the University of California at San Francisco indicates that estrogen stabilizes the heat-regulating centers in the brain. Although not completely certain, scientists believe hot flashes occur when your body temperature control center, located in the hypothalamus, becomes imbalanced. Once this thermostat is affected—probably as a result of hormonal fluctuation—your ability to adjust body temperature is thrown off. The result is a hot flash followed by a hot flush. Hot flush? Technically speaking, some doctors make a distinction between a flash and a flush. They define a flash as a sense of oncoming warmth that acts as a kind of warning signal. A flush—what we usually think of when we use the term *hot flash*—is a deep blushing of your upper body, with heat emanating from your upper chest into your neck, face, and arms. Your skin actually reddens and increases in temperature by as much as seven degrees, your pulse speeds up, and you break out in a sweat. Flash or flush, they are both hot, and to make it simple, *hot flash* will be used to describe both phenomena.

Many women also experience a brief cold flash after a hot one. They actually feel chilled and often need to put on layers they have just finished shedding in order to be comfortable. It is similar to feeling cold after a strenuous walk during which you may have worked up a sweat, taken off your jacket, cooled off, and then found yourself getting chilly. Researchers attribute this short, rapid cool-down to the body's natural effort to regulate temperature.

My hot flashes weren't so severe that I was uncomfortable or dying. But they were warm enough to almost feel sensual, especially with a sort of cooling-off period when they were over. I never felt they were unbearable. Frankly, I was so involved in my work with students and teaching that when I got a hot flash, I just mopped my brow, fanned myself, and moved on. I've never been awakened by any, unlike some of my friends who have terrible night sweats and have to stick their toes out from under the blankets. They're just not that bad for me.

Single woman, 48

The Statistics

To most women just beginning perimenopause, the concept of hot flashes brings on feelings of fear and anxiety, usually based on terrible war stories passed on by other women. Some women do have severe and lengthy experiences with hot flashes, but they are not representative of most women. Here are some facts and figures to give you a more balanced view.

The truth of the matter is that while most women experience hot flashes, only 10 to 15 percent find them debilitating. Eighty percent of women who have hot flashes will experience them for more than a year, but only 25 percent of them will continue to have them for more than five years.

Then there is the weight advantage. Yes, there are some benefits to being overweight. It seems that heavier women tend to have fewer hot flashes than thin ones. This may be a result of the higher levels of estrogen stored in the fatty tissue of heavy women.

Women who exercise regularly are less likely to experience hot flashes. In a recent Swedish study of how regular physical exercise affects hot flashes and sweating, 49 percent of the physically active women had no symptoms as compared to 41 percent who did not exercise regularly.

Smokers get singled out again. It appears they tend to have more difficulty with hot flashes, probably because smoking affects the hormonal output of the ovaries.

The Real Problems and How to Handle Them

Silk shirts with underarm stains? Damp sheets and nightclothes? Afraid to wear a turtleneck? Sweating in a restaurant with new friends? While distressing, these are not insurmountable problems. You will find the real problems related to hot flashes are more insidious and stem from attitude, sleep deprivation, and emotional health.

Attitude. Even without firsthand knowledge, you have heard enough about hot flashes to imagine what they are like and sympathize with other women. However, where do you stand when it comes to sweating in public? Certainly not a moral issue, this is a question of your attitude toward unpredictable behavior and loss of control, because that is exactly what happens when you have hot flashes.

My first flash made me laugh when I finally figured out what it was. The second one still seemed fascinating and held my interest. From the third one on, however, it became a challenge. Seeing if anyone could tell that I was "flashing" became a concern, as did wearing layers of clothes and carrying a handkerchief all the time. My husband still threatens to buy a two-zone electric blanket for our bed just to keep from freezing all night, and dinner guests finally stopped asking, "Is it cold in here?"

Although you may not feel in control of your body, you do have some options as to how to respond to what is happening: whether to behave like a victim, go through the woe-is-me routine, and dwell on your discomfort and embarrassment or to take charge, determine how much this really affects your daily routine, and figure out how to handle it.

Spend some time analyzing what concerns you most about hot flashes. It may be fear of people noticing them, worry over soiled clothing, embarrassment about appearing distracted and out of sorts, or just getting hot and sweaty without any warning. Now test your concerns. Do other people actually know you are having a hot flash? Can they really tell? Certainly you can handle issues related to clothing. However, you probably will not be able to predict when your next flash may occur. Try to keep track and see if there is a pattern or if specific foods or even room temperature changes bring them on.

Take charge. You cannot make hot flashes disappear without some kind of intervention, but you can adjust your attitude in response to them.

Sleep Deprivation. There is no question that you can lose sleep over hot flashes. The version that keeps you awake half the night tossing and turning in a damp bed is also called *night sweats.* Many women wake up during the night bathed in sweat, try to cool down with a cold facial rinse, and even change nightclothes. They fall back to sleep, but they cannot recapture the sleep they have lost.

Sleep requirements are different for everyone, and sleep loss seems to affect some people more than others. So what is the problem with a little sleep loss? Depending on how you respond to a series of interrupted night's sleep, you may lose your ability to concentrate, become irritable, have trouble remembering things, and suffer from fatigue and muscle aches and pains—all in all, not a pretty picture.

> *One night I woke up and had to change my nightgown twice. The sheets were soaking wet. It was terrible. My hot flashes happened mostly at nighttime, not during the day. But the problem was I just couldn't sleep. When you don't sleep, you can't cope. And when you can't cope, you fly off the handle. That's when you turn into a shrew.*
>
> Married mother, 51

Short of undergoing drug or alternative therapy to alleviate hot flashes entirely (see Chapter 4, "Hormone Replacement Therapy," and Chapter 5, "Alternative Treatment"), the next logical step is to try to get more sleep by doing something to get through the continual nighttime awakenings. Several simple solutions probably come to mind—sleeping pills, an earlier bedtime, some brandy late in the evening—none of which really works. Instead, sleep experts recommend the following.

- *Keep a sleep chart.* One of the keys to a good night's sleep is maintaining a regular schedule. This means waking up and going to sleep at around the same time each day. Because the sleep cycle is governed by your body clock, it is important to give it clear knowledge on the length of a day. Your body automatically makes this calculation by determining the interval between when you wake up on Monday morning and when you get up on Tuesday morning. It does not allow for weekends and late nights. The interval has to be regular or your body will not process the information correctly. So in order to give your body the time of day, it is essential to go to bed and wake up at about the same time every day, seven days a week.

Maintain a simple chart for a month, noting the time you go to bed each night and when you wake up in the morning. Be rigid about your sleep schedule.

If you wake up too early in the morning, try bright light exposure. This means sitting in an extremely brightly lit room for an hour before bedtime in order to adjust your wake-up time to occur a little later. The lights that move the body clock need to be very bright and as close to daylight as you can make them.

- *Stop taking drugs that affect your central nervous system, including caffeine and alcohol.* No matter how convinced you may be that caffeine and alcohol do not affect your sleep, you should take a hard look at the facts. Caffeine remains in your system for twelve to twenty hours and is perhaps the worst drug for sleep. Alcohol is not much better. Often considered the world's oldest sleeping pill, alcohol does relax you and make you drowsy. Unfortunately, these effects reverse themselves seven to ten hours later, causing restlessness and seriously impacting the quality of sleep.

  Over-the-counter drugs that act on your central nervous system, such as nasal decongestants, antiasthma pills, and diet aids, will also affect sleep. If you take any of these medications and find yourself up at night, try staying off them for a while. Nicotine acts as a stimulant to the nervous system, too, providing another reason to quit smoking.

- *Exercise and get into good physical shape.* In addition to a long list of benefits, regular and rigorous exercise will assure you of a good night's sleep. This does not mean you have to go out and run 5 miles a day. Walking just one hour a day, four or five days a week, is effective (see Chapter 6, "Nutrition and Exercise"). Do this on a regular basis and you will increase your chances of getting a good night's sleep.

- *Take a hot bath before you go to bed at night.* Raising your body temperature is a proven way to induce deeper, longer-lasting sleep. However, a hot bath may also trigger a hot flash in some women.
- *Try drinking warm malted milk, preferably low-fat or skim, at bedtime.* Yes, this sounds like Grandmother's remedy for restless nights, but British doctors recently completed a study showing its effectiveness. After a glass of warm malted milk, sleep quality was better, body movements were less, and maximum effect was achieved later on in the sleep cycle.

Emotional Health. How you feel about yourself has a significant bearing on your ability to cope with hot flashes. For example, if you tend to be insecure about your physical appearance, you will probably focus on how you look during a hot flash and live in fear that others will detect what is going on. On the other hand, if you are confident and self-assured, you will quickly come up with solutions to the problems of perspiring in public places. Awareness of your emotional strengths and weaknesses can help you gain perspective on your reaction to hot flashes. However, you still have to deal with the discomfort, frustration, and lack of control. Translated to daily living, this means that you will probably have to change the way you operate: more patience, some creativity, and an expanded sense of humor. So, get a grip on things. Remember, hot flashes do not last forever.

Help with Hormone Replacement Therapy

Hot flashes send more women to doctors in search of help than any other sign of menopause. If none of the previous recommendations suits your needs, you can take comfort in knowing that hot flashes can usually be eliminated quickly and completely with hormone replacement therapy. Although it has pluses and minuses, hormone replacement therapy works to end hot flashes for the vast majority of women. So if all else fails and your life is made miserable by these heated and unpredictable events, take heart—there is an answer to your problem (see Chapter 4, "Hormone Replacement Therapy").

I tried everything to cope with my hot flashes; I even changed the way I dressed. I no longer wore any woolen sweaters—everything became cotton. My nightgowns, my underpants, even my bra. And I'd still break out in a sweat at the most inopportune times. After a while, I just tried to grin and bear it. But nobody seemed to be suffering as badly as I. My friends were not awakened in the middle of the night and didn't have flashes anywhere near as often as I did. They would try to comfort me by saying, "It's going to pass," or "It really doesn't go on for very long." But finally, I threw in the towel and said to my doctor, "Please give me a pill and make this all go away."

Since then, I've been on hormone replacement and my hot flashes and other symptoms have disappeared. I get plenty of sleep and feel terrific.

Married mother, 56

Vaginal Dryness

Although vaginal dryness may not be a common topic of conversation among your friends, it affects the majority of women to one degree or another. It is not pleasant, most women find it embarrassing to discuss, and many suffer needlessly for long periods of time. Vaginal dryness is an indicator of menopause, and you may begin to experience it during perimenopause. More than likely, it will not become a problem for five to ten years after menopause. It is treatable, reversible in most cases, and need not plague you for the rest of your life.

To be honest, vaginal dryness was a shock. I had no idea it had anything to do with menopause. Because I have a tipped womb, my doctor always asked me if I had pain during intercourse. And I didn't until very recently. Of course, when it started to hurt, I assumed it was my tipped womb. What a surprise to find out it was menopause. Now I talk about it with my friends who have had similar experiences.

Married mother, 53

The Facts

As estrogen production decreases during perimenopause, several areas of your body are affected, including the vagina. Usually very elastic with incredible stretching ability, the vagina starts to shrink as available estrogen decreases. It becomes thinner, easier to tear, and loses some of its mucous membrane. The result? Lack of lubrication, itching and irritation, susceptibility to vaginal infections, difficult or painful intercourse, postcoital bleeding, and, in some cases, involuntary contraction of the vagina in order to prevent intercourse. Left untreated, vaginal dryness can cause constant discomfort, devastate your sex life, and seriously impact your self-esteem (see Chapter 7, "Sex").

Your Options

No laughing matter, vaginal dryness is something you can do without. This is not the time to grin and bear it. Take advantage of the various remedies to avoid this troublesome condition. Even without premenopausal levels of estrogen, you are capable of vaginal lubrication for the rest of your life.

Getting It Regularly. Simple as it may seem, one of the best cures for vaginal dryness is regular sex. This means achieving orgasm once or twice a week with a partner or by masturbation; some doctors recommend masturbation with a mechanical aid to provide maximum stimulation to the vagina. Either way, you will increase the blood flow to your vagina, stimulate the mucous membrane, and exercise the surrounding muscle.

One woman took this advice to heart and made the most of her willing partner's enthusiasm:

I'm lucky to be married to my husband . . . he loves sex. So I guess I'll never have to worry about not getting enough. I know having regular sex helps with vaginal dryness. So does he. If two or three days go by, he'll kiddingly shake his finger at me and say, "Uh-oh, vaginal dryness." Usually we both laugh and head for the bedroom.

Married mother, 51

Lubricants. Some women feel the use of a lubricant on the vagina before sex is an admission of failure, whereas others view it as a pleasurable enhancement. The real issue, especially if you have never used a lubricant, is being comfortable with the concept, making it a part of sexual foreplay, and choosing the right one.

There are several good vaginal lubricants available over-the-counter, some of which are listed below. Vaseline and baby oil are not among them because they are not water soluble. Because the menopausal vagina is less lubricated and therefore less effective in regular self-cleaning, it is more likely to become infected. Non-water-soluble lubricants do not wash off easily and tend to hang around in the vagina, making it a great breeding ground for bacteria. Try one of these instead:

- *Astroglide.* Yes, that is really the name of this product, manufactured in—where else—California. It is one of the best lubricants on the market and has no taste or smell. What's more, it is light, not gunky, gooey, or gellike. Astroglide is the closest thing to your own natural lubrication.
- *K-Y Jelly.* One of the oldest and most well-known lubricants, it is perfectly adequate for the job but definitely not on the top of the list. It is viscous and not at all natural in the way it feels. You touch it and immediately know it is not like any lubrication you ever produced when aroused.
- *Replens.* Not really a lubricant in the technical sense, Replens is actually a nonprescription moisturizer for the vagina, which you apply three or four times a week just like you would apply a face cream. It works by plumping up the tissue in the vaginal lining with moisture and has the advantage of not needing to be used just before intercourse.

- *Hormone replacement therapy and estrogen cream.* Standard dosages of hormone replacement therapy are effective for a vast majority of women, although whether the pill or patch works better is a matter of individual response. Some women complain that although their vagina is more lubricated, it is not as good as new. Working closely with your doctor on the proper dosage should solve this problem.

  Another form of hormone replacement therapy, estrogen cream is applied directly to the vagina. The dosage strength is extremely low, but delivered in very small amounts, it effectively restores the vagina and its lubricating capability. It is important to note, however, that estrogen cream carries the same risks as oral and transdermal estrogen, and the decision on its use should be given the same thoughtful consideration (see Chapter 4, "Hormone Replacement Therapy").

The reason I started taking hormones was because I knew you could become very dry and end up with painful sex. Look, I don't mind wrinkles, I don't mind growing old. But if I have to give up sex, forget it. I just won't allow that to happen and I'll do anything I can to prevent it. I'm not even interested in plastic surgery on the outside—I only want it on the inside!

Single mother, 49

Dress Right. Vaginal dryness can also lead to irritation, infection, and itching. An easy way to inhibit vaginal itching and curb the growth of bacteria, which can lead to infection, is to wear the right kind of underclothes. This means panties or pantyhose with cotton crotches, which allow air to circulate and create an unfriendly environment for bacteria.

Urinary Stress Incontinence

As scary as it might sound, urinary stress incontinence, another effect of decreasing estrogen production, is a temporary condition that can be controlled and reversed. No, you will not regress to early childhood and start to wet the bed. Nor will you need to wear rubber panties. However, you will have to face reality and do what it takes to avoid discomfort and embarrassment.

The Facts

Urinary stress incontinence is the involuntary loss of bladder control in response to sudden muscular stress. It usually occurs as a result of weakened muscles in the pelvic area. Because these muscles have estrogen receptors, they naturally lose their tone as estrogen production declines, which is just what happens during perimenopause.

The urethra, which passes urine out of the bladder, is built similarly to the vagina and responds negatively to a decreased estrogen supply. The mucous lining becomes thin, and the surrounding muscles start to weaken slightly. None of this is really noticeable until you put stress on your bladder, like coughing, laughing, or jogging. These type of movements pull at the opening of the urethra, and if the muscles are not strong enough, they will not be able to resist the tug. This results in a momentary loss of bladder control and the release of a small amount of urine.

Because there also are other causes of urinary incontinence, it is important to see a doctor for an accurate diagnosis. There is a wide variety of treatment available, from drugs to surgery, and proper diagnosis is key, especially if your incontinence goes beyond the mild form usually associated with perimenopause.

Your Options

This is not the moment to run out and buy a box of adult diapers to avoid an accident. It is time to help your body cope with the situation.

Kegel Exercises. There are exercises for your hips, thighs, arms, buttocks, and almost every other part of your body. Luckily, there are also exercises for your pelvic floor—the muscles that control your bladder, bowels, and sexual orgasm. Named for the

California surgeon who invented them in the 1950s, Dr. Arnold Kegel, they are easy, not terribly strenuous, and invisible to the rest of the world. This means you can do them while riding in a car, waiting for a meeting, watching television, or reading a book.

1. Locate your pelvic floor muscles by pretending to stop the flow of urine while urinating. You will feel a distinct tightening, and most likely you will not be able to maintain this squeeze because these muscles are weak.
2. Tighten these muscles again and release. Repeat this ten times. Because it does not seem to matter how long you squeeze, you can do these muscle contractions as quickly as you like. The important thing is to tighten and release. Do not bother to hold your breath—it will not help.
3. Repeat these series of ten muscle squeezes five to ten times each day, for a total of fifty to one hundred contractions. Anything less will not be effective.

The key to success is to make these exercises habit-forming and associate them with part of your daily routine. Brush your teeth, do your Kegels. Stop at red lights, do your Kegels. Watch the news. Blow-dry your hair. Do your Kegels. Whatever it takes, the benefits go beyond preventing an embarrassing accident. Kegels also strengthen muscles that can improve sex and relieve hemorrhoids. Think of them as a secret but powerful internal fitness program.

Hormone Replacement Therapy. Just one of the many benefits of hormone replacement therapy, estrogen seems to have a positive effect by restoring blood flow to weakened portions of the pelvic area, including the urinary tract. In order to opt for hormone replacement therapy, you will need to assess the propriety of this regimen with your doctor (see Chapter 4, "Hormone Replacement Therapy").

The Emotional Roller Coaster

It is important to set the record straight right from the start. Menopause does not cause depression. Nor does it turn you into a crazy person. Studies show that women who have recently gone through menopause did not have higher levels of depression, anxiety, or stress than women of the same age who were still menstruating. We have come a long way from the days when menopause was believed to cause insanity.

Then what is this emotional roller coaster ride all about? For some women, it just does not exist. For others, it can be a series of heightened mood swings experienced each month just before menstruation. And it is real. These moods can come on with surprising intensity and can leave you feeling as if an alien has taken over your body. Usually, this behavior is temporary and will disappear after menopause.

There is a third group of women with a history of ongoing emotional problems, including clinically diagnosed depression. The symptoms of perimenopause may exacerbate their condition. These women also tend to have more complaints about their symptoms and will probably continue to be affected until they deal with the cause of their illness.

The Facts

Mood swings and mild depression occurring one to two weeks each month before menstruation are now officially recognized by the medical community as part of PMS. Doctors believe that PMS can start or intensify in your late 30s and continue through perimenopause. The exact causes of PMS are not clear, but approximately 10 percent of all women experience it, most of whom are over 35 years old.

I always thought PMS happened to other people and never to me. Mainly because I'm so healthy and feel wonderful 99.9 percent of the time. I thought all those things I heard women complain about were just an excuse. Until I realized it was happening to me. Actually, it was my husband who noticed it first and said,

"Honey, you just aren't yourself today. What's wrong?" I couldn't put a finger on it, but I knew I felt touchy and irritable.

Married woman, 45

Other factors affecting your moods are often associated with what is going on around you. The state of your mental health is directly related to what is happening in your life. Are you going through changes such as looking for a new job, reevaluating your love life, sending kids to college, caring for aging parents, or raising a young child? Any of these life events can sap your strength and energy and leave you feeling blue, especially if you are also experiencing hormonal changes.

Your Options

Even when you can identify the cause of a sudden mood change, it is still difficult to stand back and take control. Sometimes it is like watching a runaway train—you can see it careening toward disaster but feel powerless to stop it. Perimenopause is often difficult, and you are entitled to feel down from time to time. It is a period of enormous change and unpredictability, but it will not last forever. Try to focus on the following to get through the rough times.

Self-analysis. If you have a normal emotional profile and find yourself acting cranky, feeling negative about everything, or just generally blue, stop for a moment and try to analyze what is really going on. Do these feelings last all month or just a few days? Do they seem strange and uncontrollable? Is this moodiness affecting your ability to function?

Make an attempt to separate real sources of anger and frustration from trivial annoyances that get blown out of proportion on one of your black days. Distance yourself from the situation and take a hard look at the real issues. You may find that none exist and it is just a matter of getting through a one- or two-day period of gloom. Keep an image of your usual cheery disposition in mind and try not to feel like you are turning into a monster.

Remember that these negative feelings are temporary and try to maintain a positive outlook.

On the other hand, you may realize there are some larger issues that really are bothering you. Focus on them and get angry if you need to. Many women have a hard time expressing anger and some even need a day of perimenopause crankiness to feel they have permission to let off steam.

Instead of feeling guilty and defensive about mood swings, this woman decided to own up to her hormonal changes and call a spade a spade.

We've always been an open couple, and Tom is constantly aware of my moods. If I'm not behaving like the up, happy woman he married twenty-six years ago, he always blames it on my period. It used to annoy me, but who else is going to know me as well. I live with this man. I sleep with this man, and he gets the brunt of any changes that happen with me.

I've noticed over the last couple of years that I am intent sometimes on making Tom wrong about anything just so that I can jump on him. Now that I realize what is going on, when I'm really cruel and nasty, I'll say, "It's all right, Tom, you can't win here. No matter what you do, you're 'it' today." Sometimes we even manage to joke about it and he'll say, "Oh, never mind. I know it's your hormones, and they're all screwed up today."

Married mother, 51

Diet and Exercise. This may sound like Mom-and-apple-pie advice, but paying attention to what you eat and how you exercise will guarantee an improvement in your outlook on life (see Chapter 6, "Nutrition and Exercise").

Eating foods high in sugar and caffeine can set you up for a roller coaster ride with more ups and downs than you can imagine. You know the old expression "What goes up must eventually come down." Well, that is exactly what happens to your body. Caffeine and sugar are stimulants. They take you up and help you feel more energetic and alive. When these effects wear off, just like a drug, your spirits often plummet along with your blood sugar. You can control what you eat. Make the choice to avoid adding to the emotional swings that can be brought on by perimenopause.

As for regular exercise, it is a well-known tonic for down-and-out moments. It invigorates, makes you feel good, and gives you a sense of accomplishment. Vigorous exercise can also release endorphins into your system, causing what is known as a "runner's high." Endorphins have an analgesic effect and can give you a sense of well-being—almost like taking mood-enhancing drugs with no unpleasant aftereffects. Whether you walk, run, take aerobics classes, or swim, you will find the benefits of regular exercise essential to feeling good about yourself.

Vitamins. Many people still think of vitamins as the "fruit and nuts" category of medicine, even though controlled studies have shown their effectiveness in treating various ailments. The debate about vitamins will undoubtedly continue, but many people have benefited enormously from specifically prescribed regimens.

Dr. Leo Galland, a noted PMS specialist in private practice in New York, advocates a gradual four-stage approach to treatment. If you do not respond to the first stage after about a month, another is added until you have relief from symptoms.

- *The first stage* focuses on diet, as discussed earlier in this chapter, with an emphasis on reduced intake of salt, fat, and sugar and complete avoidance of caffeine. This is difficult for some women because they experience salt and sugar cravings premenstrually.
- *The second stage* is a daily dose of B-complex vitamins that contains 50 to 100 milligrams of vitamin B_6 plus 300 milligrams of elemental magnesium. Try to find magnesium gluconate tablets, as they are most easily absorbed; you will need to take several of them in order to get the required 300 milligrams of elemental magnesium. Magnesium levels seem to be affected during PMS, and taking a supplement can be very helpful. However, too much can cause diarrhea. The recommended dose is safe and usually beneficial

for women who have premenstrual constipation.

Please note: As with any vitamin, these should be taken on a full stomach. Remember, taking more than the recommended dosage can be extremely harmful—more is not better.

- *The third stage* adds 400 to 600 international units of vitamin E. Controlled studies of magnesium, vitamin B_6, and vitamin E have shown that each has an effect on PMS. Vitamin E is also known to give some women relief from mild hot flashes.

- *The fourth stage* has two options, both of which are a source of essential fatty acids: either flax oil, 1 tablespoon daily, or evening primrose oil, six capsules daily. Research has shown evening primrose oil to be effective in relieving premenstrual breast tenderness and pain; it is also effective in treating mild hot flashes. Because evidence suggests that evening primrose oil has an estrogenic effect, women with a sensitivity to estrogen, especially those with a history of breast cancer or migraine headaches, should use it with caution.

Although it is unlikely that the above recommendations will harm you, it is always smart to consult a health practitioner before ingesting any substances, natural or otherwise. Be open-minded and give it a try.

Headaches, Crawling Skin, and Memory Loss

Although the most common complaints of women experiencing perimenopause focus on sleep loss, mood swings, hot flashes, irregular periods, vaginal dryness, and incontinence, there are several other menopausal indicators worth mentioning. Experienced by a small percentage of women, certain kinds of headaches; crawling skin (formication); and memory loss also seem to be associated with perimenopause. You may not be next in line for any of these symptoms, but it helps to know about them, understand they are temporary, and be comforted that they usually disappear after menopause.

Headaches

> *I have really bad headaches with my period. It can be a few days before or a few days after and sometimes it happens when I'm ovulating. Luckily, I'm able to feel comfortable with a couple of extra-strength Tylenol. But I don't want to keep taking them. My periods stopped for about seven months and the headaches went away, too. Then all of a sudden, I got this whopper migraine, and sure enough, a couple of days later my period started again.*
>
> Single woman, 44

Women who suffer from headaches and tend to experience them one to two weeks before menstruating are now being diagnosed as having menstrual migraine. This syndrome affects at least 60 percent of women with migraine headaches and, because of the close association with menstruation, is considered to be hormonally related. New neuroendocrine studies show that migraine sufferers may be sensitive to fluctuating estrogen levels, which often act as a migraine trigger prior to menstruation. Some women stop having headaches after menopause, whereas others report an increase. Unfortunately, it is impossible to predict.

Menstrual migraine headaches are sometimes triggered by sex hormones either occurring naturally or taken as supplements. More often, certain foods, alcohol, irregular eating and sleeping habits, or excessive stress can also bring one on. They usually occur just before monthly menstruation, midway through bleeding, or at ovulation. Women with menstrual migraines may also have monthly breast tenderness and water retention.

If you suffer from these headaches, there are a few things you can do to lessen your chances of bringing one one. Try to isolate specific factors that might trigger a headache by keeping a record both of your headaches and your menstrual cycle. It is important to note your behavior pattern in relation to each headache. This means recording potential headache triggers mentioned earlier, including food, alcohol, stress levels, and sleep habits. In this way you may be able to identify just what sets off your headaches.

Exercise also seems to have a positive effect as does sexual activity. If you have menstrual migraines and take hormone replacement therapy as well, you should investigate trying another brand of hormones, as this may be beneficial. If nothing else works, anti-inflammatory drugs like Advil and Nuprin will give you some relief.

Crawling Skin (Formication)

This may sound like something out of a Stephen King novel, but the creepy, crawly feeling some women experience during perimenopause is not a work of fiction. It can seem like there are little invisible critters running relay races on your arms and legs or feel like constant tingling or numbness.

Crawling skin is not a widespread phenomenon, but the women who experience formication (an itchy sensation, as if tiny insects were crawling on the skin) complain about it sometime during the twelve months after their last period. Although not fully documented, formication does respond to estrogen therapy. Homeopathic remedies containing sepia (squid ink) may also have a positive effect. The medical community still does not know much about formication; fortunately, the symptoms usually disappear within a year.

Memory Loss

This is the real scary stuff. You go upstairs to get something you need and forget what it is by the time you get to the top landing. Or you excitedly tell a friend about the two movies you saw over the weekend and cannot come up with the name of the second one. What is happening here? Are you going to lose all your marbles before you reach 60? Hardly, but memory lapses like these are disconcerting and can affect your self-confidence.

It is not uncommon for both men and women to experience this kind of short-term memory loss, especially in their middle years, but women seem to be distressed by it more. Unfortunately, only limited research has been done to determine if this short-term memory loss in women is directly related to decreasing estrogen levels during perimenopause. In a small eight-month study of fifty women with surgical menopause, those who opted for hormone replacement therapy scored higher on tests of short- and long-term memory than those who received a placebo, no matter what mood the women were in at the time. This suggests that estrogen production can affect memory in women with surgical menopause. It also questions the long-standing idea that memory loss is linked to depression. However, the women who did not receive hormones were still able to function quite well, and their performance at work and home was not impaired.

Although the results of this study cannot be extrapolated to all women going through menopause, the following list of brain facts will give you some perspective on memory, intelligence, and aging:

- Although the makeup of the brain changes with age, your intelligence does not decrease. If you were a whiz kid in your teens, you will be just as bright, or maybe even smarter, in your 80s.
- Brain performance, including memory, can be affected by high blood pressure, vitamin deficiencies, overmedication, drug or drug–food interactions, malnutrition, anemia, sleep loss, or stress.
- Short-term memory loss experienced by some women during perimenopause is temporary and seems to disappear after menopause. However, if memory loss persists after menopause, you should discuss it with your doctor.
- After the age of 65, only 5 to 7 percent of women and men show serious intellectual impairment.
- Older people remember almost as much as their younger counterparts, but it often takes their brains longer to retrieve the data.

Being able to see the humor in some of your memory lapses can make all the difference, as it did for this menopausal woman.

I have a fantastic memory; I've always loved my memory. And up until recently, I never had to have a list to keep track of things. But this short-term memory loss I've been having recently is enough to make you crazy. I'm getting to be like everyone else I know who is always forgetting things. At work, I forgot where I put the wastepaper basket and wasted fifteen minutes looking until I found it. Then there was the time I lost my pen, only to discover I had been using it to stir my tea. It's turned into a joke at this point, but I really wish my memory would get back to where it used to be.

Married woman, 53

Given the available information on menopause and memory loss, it is likely that your moments of forgetfulness are related to lack of sleep, stress, or part of the aging process. One way to deal with these lapses is not to panic and to accept them as just that. Assume that your brain definitely has the knowledge at hand and that it might take a little bit longer to retrieve. Once you become more relaxed about this little glitch in your brain waves, you will find that by reducing the added stress you create with fear of not remembering, your memory capability actually improves. It is almost a matter of self-confidence: If you are convinced that you will remember what you seem to have forgotten sooner or later, then it is bound to happen.

Nevertheless, if memory loss is really creating havoc in your life, you should seek medical advice. Otherwise, make extra lists, use some of the tried-and-true mnemonic tricks to remember things, and always have a pen and paper at the ready.

False Alarms

Once you become reconciled to some of the changes affecting your body during perimenopause, you will probably want it all to hurry up and be over. This kind of wishful thinking sets you up for the big come-on—two, six, maybe even eight months without your period. You start to enjoy the freedom and are convinced you are finally going to experience menopause. Then all of a sudden you get your period again and feel like you are right back at square one. You were ready for the change, it turned out to be nothing more than a false alarm, and you are left feeling angry and frustrated.

This woman's experience is more common than you might think.

I was concerned at first when my period stopped. I had no idea what was happening to my body and I didn't know if it was normal, especially because I was only 43. After I saw a doctor, I realized it was all right. Menopause is just a part of the natural progression of life. I was really happy that I wouldn't have to mess around with my period anymore. And then, seven months later, my period started again and I got angry that it was back. I felt cheated out of the freedom I had gotten used to. So I'm anxious for menopause to happen.

Married mother, 45

Take small comfort in the fact that you are not alone. Missing your period for several months only to have it resume is common, especially if you are under 50 years old. In fact, if you are between 45 and 49 and have not menstruated for up to seven months, there is a 50 percent chance that you will start to menstruate again.

You will become a full-fledged member of the club and experience menopause sooner or later. Perimenopause, with all its ups and downs, will then be behind you.

Chapter Three

Postmenopause

I'm too old to be young and too young to be old.
—Evelyn Couch,
Fried Green Tomatoes

It is probably difficult to think of yourself as postmenopausal, but in medical terms, this is an appropriate description of a woman who has experienced menopause. This means you have not had your period for more than a year and your body is adjusting to significantly smaller amounts of available estrogen. By definition, you will remain postmenopausal for the rest of your life, regardless of whether or not you take hormone replacement therapy.

It sounds a lot like a lifetime sentence for bad behavior, but *postmenopause* is just a word used to identify the reproductive stage of your body as you get older. It is not a word used to describe your lifestyle or how you look and feel, nor is it a label. It certainly does not reflect the new sense of freedom and energy most women feel in their middle years. We need to come up with a different word that more accurately describes this phase of life, one that sounds less clinical and more positive. Until then, postmenopause will have to do.

A good example of refusing to be labeled anything is the

strategy of this active woman in her late 40s. Although still in perimenopause, she managed to avoid being tainted by negative impressions of menopause. She observed enough positive actions on the part of her menopausal friends to feel all right about the prospect of her own approaching menopause.

> I really think that you have to be positive about this whole menopausal thing. You can't stop it—it's just something you have to go through. Sure, some women have it harder than others, but then again, some women get their periods easily and some don't. I just think it's your outlook that's important. Menopause is not the end; it's the beginning of something else. And when you see women who are in their early 50s who have a positive attitude, they look fabulous. They seem to be so much more aware of what is going on. At my reunion, the women who stayed up until 3:00 in the morning were all between the ages of 45 and 55, and they were dancing with all the younger men who were dying to get out on the dance floor and have fun. It was all part of having a positive attitude.
>
> Married mother, 49

There are many issues associated with postmenopause—some health related and others focused on physical appearance. Although postmenopause continues through old age, this chapter will concentrate on those issues especially important during the first fifteen years. As your body changes after menopause, you will need to reckon with the possibility of medical problems like osteoporosis, heart disease, and diabetes. You will also have to come to terms with more obvious physical changes like wrinkles and unwanted hair.

Middle age is not for sissies. So get a grip, be informed, and take some action to make the most of these fruitful years.

Osteoporosis

> Up until age 44, I had led a charmed life with no significant physical ailments. Then early one morning, while leisurely walking

to the corner store, I tripped on a huge crack in the sidewalk and ended up in the emergency room with a broken baby finger on my right hand and an amputated nail on the ring finger of my left. No big deal, right? Wrong. Four weeks in a cast up to my elbow instantly taught me humility. After an initial week of severe pain and feelings that ran the gamut from fear and self-pity to anger and frustration, I began to live life temporarily crippled. I couldn't write, pull up my pants, cook, use a tampon, dry my hair, or drive my standard-shift car. Lucky for me, it was all over in six weeks and I was back to my daily routine. Determined, fiercely independent, and with the help of family and many friends, I managed to get along all right during that time. I also learned I wasn't invincible and that a broken bone is a very serious and far-reaching injury.

Married mother, 46

Imagine breaking a bone under different circumstances. Instead of being 44, physically fit, and in good health, you are 68, with poor vision, seldom-exercised muscles, a heart condition, and a tendency toward clumsiness. You fall and fracture your hip. Not only will you suffer extreme pain and discomfort, you will also have to undergo major surgery to repair your hip. Given your physical condition, you are probably not the best candidate for this kind of operation, but it is unlikely you will ever regain full use of your joint without it. This could mean a significant loss of self-reliance and, depending on your circumstances, require full-time care in a nursing home. In fact, less than 50 percent of people who have a hip fracture ever get back to a lifestyle similar to what they had; 25 percent of them will end up in walkers, wheelchairs, and pain.

What about shrinking from a height of 5'5" to 5'2"? This might not sound so terrible, but loss of body height may be directly related to fractures of the vertebrae. With this shrinking comes distortion of your spine's normal curves and even just a few vertebral fractures can cause you to develop a dowager's hump and protruding abdomen, with your ribs practically sitting on your pelvis.

Osteoporosis is insidious. Most of the time it goes undetected until a fracture occurs, and by then, it is usually too late to reverse the condition. It is imperative that you understand the worst things that can happen as a result of osteoporosis and be motivated enough to do what it takes to prevent them.

Most women still feel strong and at the top of their game when they first reach menopause. Perhaps this is why it is so hard to imagine yourself ravaged by the effects of time. However, the changes in your body as you enter postmenopause are dramatic. They can happen quickly but silently, and you must pay attention right away. Right now.

The Facts

Osteoporosis is defined as a condition of porous bones and usually occurs as a result of the loss of bone mass. This means that there is just too little of it to do the job, and what bone exists may not be up to snuff. Like all high-quality structural material, bones are designed to be strong, support weight, and stand up to trauma from outside forces. However, osteoporotic bone looks more like a honeycomb, breaks easily, and barely supports the weight of your body.

First, a little about bones in general. Formed in a variety of shapes and sizes, bones are the framework of your body, protect vital organs, act as a reservoir for calcium, and heal after breaking. You might expect all bone to be thick and dense, but in fact, although 80 percent is compact bone, the remaining 20 percent, called *trabecular bone,* is spongelike in structure and not nearly as dense. Trabecular bone is found in the irregular-shaped parts of the skeleton such as the spine, pelvis, and at the ends of bones, near the joints.

In a form of preventive maintenance, bones remain strong by remodeling themselves on a continuous basis—older bone is replaced by newer, stronger bone. During childhood and adolescence, the amount of new bone formed is greater than what is taken away. By the time you are in your 30s, the replacement balance is pretty even. When you reach your 40s, however, the balance shifts—less new bone is formed while the old bone is still taken away. This depletion also happens unevenly and you lose more trabecular than compact bone. Bone mass loss continues gradually until you are about 80. Unless you are a woman. Then you get the double whammy: bone loss from both aging and lack of estrogen.

For eight to ten years after menopause, the lack of estrogen accelerates bone loss and you can lose as much as 3 to 6 percent a year. It can be even worse for women who experience surgical or chemically induced menopause because the estrogen supply is cut off so abruptly. In either case, according to a 1991 special report on osteoporosis by the *Harvard Health Letter*, menopause may be responsible for the loss of as much as 10 to 15 percent of a woman's compact bone mass and 15 to 30 percent of her trabecular bone mass. Add that to the effects of aging, and you come up with a total loss of up to 35 percent of compact and 50 percent of trabecular bone during a woman's lifetime.

Who Is at Risk?
This seems to be the question of the hour. Although only 25 to 30 percent of women actually develop osteoporosis, we do not know who they will be. However, we do know that all women experience an accelerated rate of bone loss after menopause. Furthermore, for a variety of reasons, many women reach menopause with a bone loss deficit and

- May never have achieved peak bone mass earlier in life—it is only in the first three decades that you get your bone mass endowment—due to diet, exercise, irregular menstrual cycles, drugs, genetics, and body type.
- May start with good bone mass and then lose it through metabolic bone disease, hyperparathyroidism, or changes in renal function.

Many women go through life without adequate bone mineral and never develop fractures, but those with weaker bones are predisposed to a higher fracture risk. Other factors such as your overall health and muscle tone play an important part in the likelihood of your sustaining an injury.

Clearly some women are more probable candidates than others. The easiest way to determine your potential for developing osteoporosis is to see which of these risk factors applies to you.

Lightweight and White. It seems that this group of women, including Asians, is prone to osteoporosis. White women have a lower bone density than blacks by as much as 5 to 10 percent. They are at a disadvantage by having a lower bone density level to start and, as they get older, simply cannot afford to lose more bone without putting themselves at risk.

Weight is also a factor. It is time to bury the second half of the old saying "You can never be too rich or too thin." Being too thin can be harmful to your health. Although the reasons are not completely understood, it seems that even a slight excess of fat has a positive effect on bone mass. It appears that estrogen is converted and stored in fat tissue more efficiently if a woman is not too skinny.

Sedentary Lifestyle. Bones are peculiar in that they respond positively to mechanical stress and strain, which stimulate them and generate growth. Exercise, especially the weight-bearing kind such as jogging, walking, and tennis, helps to keep the bone remodeling process in action. By spending your spare time in front of the television or just sitting around, you are more likely to lose a larger percentage of bone mass than if you exercise regularly.

Low-Calcium Diet. Unfortunately, this applies to most Americans. Remember how your mother nagged you to drink all your milk? Well, she was right. Unless you grew up drinking three glasses a day or popped calcium supplements on a regular basis, you probably have less bone mass than you should. There are plenty of calcium-rich foods available (see Chapter 6, "Nutrition and Exercise"), but very few of us are conscious of making them a standard part of our diet.

Smoking and Drinking. The accusing finger always seems to point in this direction. Although excessive drinking and smoking are generally bad for your health, these habits seem to have a specific negative impact on bone formation. There is no question that smokers have a higher rate of vertebral fractures, and drinkers usually eat poorly and have a greater tendency to trip and fall. Smoking appears to decrease the body's ability to convert and store estrogen, and alcohol can decrease calcium absorption as well as vitamin D synthesis and is directly toxic to bone.

Amenorrhea. Once they have started menstruating on a regular basis, some women then stop for a variety of reasons, not including pregnancy. This cessation of menses is called *amenorrhea* and can lead to bone loss. It is common among women athletes and those who suffer from anorexia nervosa. Amenorrhea is a sign that ovulation is not occurring, and therefore, estrogen, a key factor in bone maintenance, is being produced in inadequate amounts. Any woman who has stopped menstruating for six months or more at any time during her life has suffered bone loss to some degree.

Genetics. Like mother, like daughter. If osteoporosis runs in your family, there is probably a good reason. Although a hereditary gene has yet to be isolated, factors such as body type, diet, and exercise habits are passed from one generation to the next. You may not actually share the same gene pool with someone in your family who has osteoporosis, but you are likely to inherit similar lifestyle patterns, which can contribute to poor bone health. Be aware of osteoporosis in your family.

Steroid Medication. Glucocorticoid steroid therapy—not to be confused with anabolic steroids used by some athletes to build muscle—is used to treat a number of diseases such as rheumatoid arthritis, chronic active hepatitis, inflammatory bowel disease, asthma, psoriasis, and chronic pulmonary disease. Unfortunately, commonly prescribed steroids like cortisone and prednisone are known to be destructive to bones because they encourage bone loss in many different ways. Glucocorticoids upset the balance of bone remodeling and cause more bone to be taken away than is replaced. They also cause the kidneys to excrete more calcium and decrease the efficiency of calcium absorption from the intestines. All of this contributes to the risk of osteoporosis. The most important factor is the cumulative dose of these steroids over time, as lost bone is usually not replaced in adults. Most physicians who prescribe steroids are trying to limit the dose and encourage patients to take supplemental calcium. For patients who require long-term steroid treatment, the new drug deflazacort, which retains the advantages of prednisone and seems to cause less bone loss, is in clinical trials and may be available in a few years. Until then, if you take glucocorticoids, you should discuss your increased risk of osteoporosis with your doctor.

Although risk factors cannot clearly point to exactly who is going to get osteoporosis, they can provide you with advance warning about where you stand. With knowledge about her own risk profile, this woman is moving in the right direction in terms of dealing with osteoporosis.

Osteoporosis is one of the main issues concerning me about menopause. I'm part of the population that is prone to it. I'm fairly slim and small boned and hate milk, and I haven't been able to give up smoking. What's more, I may not be able to tolerate hormone replacement therapy. So I have all these things working against me, and that's really scary. I even took up lifting free weights because of my fear of osteoporosis.

Single mother, 47

Bone Density Screening

Because there is currently no cure for osteoporosis, the emphasis for fighting this condition is on prevention. This means that in addition to appropriate diet and exercise, evaluation of your current skeletal health is of primary importance. Given the fact that basic risk for osteoporosis comes down to two factors— either you do not have enough bone mass to begin with or you have a "leak" and are losing it—it makes sense to determine your skeletal status. There is no way to tell what is really going on without some sort of diagnostic test.

Fortunately, testing can be done easily and painlessly with X-ray equipment designed to measure your bone mass density. One approach is to establish a baseline bone mass measurement just before you reach menopause. Then test that against another measurement taken a year after you pass menopause. Any significant decrease will be a warning sign of your vulnerability to osteoporosis. It will show up early, and you will have time to do something about it.

Just as women should routinely have mammograms to detect abnormalities in an effort to guard against breast cancer, they should also consider bone density testing to guard against osteoporosis. This is not an obscure procedure manufactured by the medical community to make more money. Bone density screening is a proven technique for establishing bone mineral levels. According to Dr. Richard Bockman, chief of endocrinology at the Hospital for Special Surgery in New York, "As a determinant of risk, the measurement of bone mineral mass is a better predictor of those people who are going to fracture than is blood pressure a predictor of people who are going to have a stroke or blood cholesterol as a predictor of people who are going to have a heart attack. Of those kinds of tools that we as physicians use to identify the patients at risk, measurement of bone density is a better predictor."

As women become more educated on menopause and the attendant long-term health implications, the popularity of bone density testing will increase significantly. With the large numbers of women entering midlife, it is possible that bone density testing will become a routine menopausal screen, and perhaps the rate of osteoporosis will decrease.

There are very specific reasons to monitor your bone density, according to Theresa Galsworthy, R.N., director of the Osteoporosis Center at the Hospital for Special Surgery:

- To provide baseline data.
- To provide information that will determine whether patients need a bone maintenance program or additional medical evaluation and treatment.
- To assist physicians and their patients in decision making regarding estrogen replacement.
- To determine if peak bone mass is present in high-risk patients under 30 years of age.
- To provide serial testing in order to determine the efficacy of bone maintenance techniques or treatment.

This woman's experience with bone mass testing is a good example of how you can use the results to make better-informed decisions about your midlife health care.

Up until a month ago, my bone density was perfectly fine. I'd had a reading last year and was in the ninety-ninth percentile, which meant I was not in danger of fracture. This time my bone density has dropped to the eightieth percentile, which means that I'm more vulnerable to fracture. At this point, especially with my bone health heading south, I'm going to reassess taking estrogen, which I know will make a difference and perhaps stabilize my bone loss. At least with these tests, you know what is happening and can then figure out what to do about it.

Married woman, 58

Several different methods can be used for bone density testing, all of which involve relatively low-dose X-ray procedures. Listed below are the various techniques, what they measure, radiation dose, and estimated cost.

TECHNIQUE	SITE	EXAMINATION TIME (MIN)	DOSE OF RADIATION[a] (MREM)	APPROXIMATE COST
Radiographic absorptiometry (RA)	Hand	3–5	100	$75–$150
Single-photon absorptiometry (SPA)	Arm, heel	15	10–20	$75–$150
Dual-energy photon absorptiometry (DPA)	Spine, hip, total body	20–40	5	$150–$200
Dual-energy X-ray absorptiometry (DXA)	Spine, hip total body	3–7	1–3	$150–$200
Quantitative computerized tomography (QCT)	Spine	10–15	200	$150–$250

Source: National Osteoporosis Foundation.
[a] One chest X ray gives a radiation dose of 20–50 mrem; a full dental X ray, 300 mrem; and an abdominal CT (computerized tomography), 1–6 mrem.

The most popular test is either of the dual-energy techniques listed in the table. They are the most accurate technology to date and only require low doses of radiation. The SPA test is fine for measuring bone density of the arm and heel but is not helpful in predicting vertebral or hip fractures.

Bone density testing is currently available in most major cities. Large hospitals often have the necessary equipment, and some of them even have special osteoporosis centers. There is also a trend toward the establishment of satellite facilities, subsidiaries of their larger counterparts, located in smaller suburban areas and with similar equipment.

As simple as all of this sounds, there are a few pointers to keep in mind about this kind of testing:

- Make sure you use a facility that does bone density testing on a regular basis. Usually the more a technique is used, the better the quality, accuracy, and maintenance of the equipment. Choose a facility with the best available equipment, preferably DXA third-generation machinery.
- It is critical to have both a skilled technician operating the equipment and a qualified doctor or radiologist to interpret the results. Professionals at this level will be able to rule out factors that may interfere with the accuracy of test results, such as poor patient positioning or underlying bone disease.
- Try to arrange for a thorough consultation with a qualified medical professional, preferably one who specializes in metabolic bone disease, to discuss your test results and the various measures you can employ to best determine optimal bone health. A simple evaluation that your bone density is average or above average is not sufficient.
- Understand your personal commitment to this testing procedure. Unless you are prepared to act on the results of the testing, you are wasting time and money.

Already a victim of osteoporosis, this woman has taken advantage of bone density testing not only to control and monitor her condition but also to gain some peace of mind about her long-term health.

I have osteoporosis and think I'll probably be all right. I'm being monitored on a regular basis by excellent doctors. But I still feel responsible. At this point, I don't wait for the doctor to tell me how I'm doing. I can tell myself because I work on it by exercising, eating right, and having bone density tests. I have a new sense of freedom and I no longer worry about walking down the street and having my hip give way.

Married mother, 57

Unfortunately, screening for osteoporosis remains a controversial issue. Most insurance companies will only cover the cost of single-photon testing, and some doctors feel it is wasteful to test an entire female population when only 25 to 30 percent is at risk. As with anything new, controversy reigns, and ignorance about the application of bone density testing has led to a fear that it will be prescribed indiscriminately. However, enormous pressure is being brought to bear in Washington and policies regarding insurance coverage are bound to change within the next few years.

So far, however, change has been slow. Sandra Raymond, executive director of the National Osteoporosis Foundation, voices the frustration of many advocates of bone density testing. "It has been seven years that the government has been considering this technology, which all the scientific thought leaders believe to be accurate, precise, and predictive of future fractures. In the ten years it will take to finally issue a policy, there will be a decade of fractures that were needless and might have been prevented."

Specifically, the National Osteoporosis Foundation is working on establishing strict supportable guidelines for testing and insurance coverage, as stated in a report from their Scientific Advisory Board published in the *Journal of Bone and Mineral Research* in November 1989. As stated, insurance-covered bone density testing should be appropriate

- *In estrogen-deficient women,* to diagnose significantly low bone mass in order to make decisions about hormone replacement therapy.
- *In patients with vertebral abnormalities,* to diagnose spinal osteoporosis in order to make decisions about further diagnostic evaluation and therapy.
- *In patients receiving long-term glucocorticoid therapy,* to diagnose low bone mass in order to adjust therapy.
- *In patients with primary asymptomatic hyperparathyroidism,* to diagnose low bone mass in order to identify those at risk of severe skeletal disease who may be candidates for surgical intervention.

Without the imprimatur of the federal government on this technology, many private insurers will wait for a definitive statement before extending coverage to bone density testing. As head of this country's primary osteoporosis advocacy group, Ms. Raymond feels strongly that the government is abrogating its leadership role both in terms of providing public health information and funding the research that is necessary to overcome what is essentially a preventable and treatable disease. She states emphatically, "You can't say that about many of the diseases we have to deal with today. So when you've got one, like osteoporosis, that you can correct and overcome with a minimum amount of money, you should allocate the funds. Simply put, there is no government focus on prevention."

Your Options
Although there is no known way to reverse extensive bone loss once it has occurred, there are effective interventions that can prevent or minimize the seriousness of osteoporosis. Consider them carefully, be honest about your lifestyle and health, and, working with a physician, develop a course of action that will be appropriate for you.

Size Up Your Skeleton. Take a close look at the risk factors mentioned earlier and ask yourself some hard questions. How healthy were you as a young child? Did you drink milk? What about physical activity? Did you play actively as a kid and manage to make exercise part of your adult routine? Are you always on a diet, skipping meals or focusing on a single type of food? Are you thin? How many drinks do you have a day? Have you missed your periods a lot? Do you smoke? Is your mother getting shorter?

By answering these questions, you will get a sense of your risk for osteoporosis. If even a small amount of risk exists, you may want to give some serious thought to taking a bone density test.

Do Your Daily Exercise. By the time you reach 40, it is obvious that exercise is no longer optional. Usually this revelation is inspired by a desire to keep your figure, look respectable in a swimsuit, or just feel better all around. Now that you understand a little about osteoporosis, you have a new and even stronger reason to exercise. Remember, bones respond well to stress and strain. Not only will the rigor of a daily physical routine promote the remodeling process, it will also tip the scales in favor of more bone made and less bone lost.

Weight-bearing exercise is the key to creating this positive stress on your bones and includes walking, jogging, aerobics, dancing, stair-climbing machines, tennis, and just about anything that keeps your feet planted on the ground. Swimming and biking are less advantageous for positive bone stress, but the muscle tone they help create is essential in preventing injury from tripping or falling. Research shows that just three hours a week of weight-bearing exercise can decrease bone loss by as much as 75 percent, and women who work out regularly have a bone density that is often 10 percent higher than that of women who do not. Regular exercise seems like more than a reasonable option and one that is totally beneficial (see Chapter 6, "Nutrition and Exercise").

Exercise may not be your idea of fun, but here is how a woman faced with the reality of osteoporosis changed her attitude.

The results of my bone density tests indicated that I had osteoporosis and my bones were like those of a much older person. So one of the things my doctor recommended was exercise, either jogging or race walking. I tried race walking and even took a class to get the rhythm right, but I hated it. The motions were hard for me and I felt sluggish. Meanwhile all sorts of people kept running past me and I started to get the jogging bug. I started by walking and jogging until I got up to about a mile and a half. Now I try to jog every day and run about 3 or 4 miles. I may not make world-class time, but I finish. It isn't really that hard and I know I have to do it for my health. Now I'm caught up in it and feel great. My doctor says energy begets energy. He's right. I have long, productive days and I love it.

Single woman, 59

Investigate Your Eating Habits. Americans are not known for their stellar eating habits. Too much fat, too much salt, too much protein. It is just this kind of gastronomical behavior that affects your ability to absorb calcium, critical for bone health, and increases your risk for osteoporosis.

Take protein, for example. Studies have shown that excess protein, which is not stored by the body, increases the amount of urinary calcium excreted through the kidneys, thus decreasing the amount of calcium absorption. Proof positive, vegetarians are known to have higher bone density measurement than omnivores.

Sodium, sugar, and caffeine, not known for their contribution to good nutrition, also promote the excretion of calcium in the urine. Alcohol is not much better. Three drinks a day is all it takes to put you at greater risk for osteoporosis. Behind the scenes, alcohol is directly toxic to bone-forming cells and may interfere with calcium absorption by affecting the cells lining the intestines. It may also interfere with the liver's ability to synthesize vitamin D.

Another culprit is phosphorus, a mineral necessary to metabolize calcium. Most people get too much of a good thing by eating excessive quantities of red meat, white bread, processed cheese, and soft drinks. A surfeit of phosphorus actually accelerates bone demineralization and increases urinary calcium levels. So as a rule of thumb, avoid consuming large quantities of foods with ingredient labels that include sodium phosphate, potassium phosphate, phosphoric acid, pyrophosphate, or polyphosphate.

Examine Your Calcium and Vitamin Intake Even with all the publicity about osteoporosis and the importance of a diet rich in calcium, more than 75 percent of women get less than 800 milligrams of calcium a day and 25 percent of them take in less than 300 milligrams. What is the recommended daily requirement?

There is no question that you need a lot of calcium growing up, while your bones are still forming and your skeleton is growing. Doctors also believe calcium is important for older people, whose physiological function is probably not as efficient as it used to be. After all, your bones are primarily made up of calcium and need it to maintain strength. According to Dr. Bockman, "If you're going to build and maintain your bone mass, you need calcium—there's no way around it, even if you're taking estrogen." Studies have borne out the need for calcium very clearly. Time and again it has been proven that women who ingest an inadequate amount of calcium will have lower bone mass than those women who take in an adequate amount. Calcium definitely prevents bone loss, and because it is not usually harmful, recommended intake for women in their middle years has increased significantly.

Opinions are varied among doctors about the precise amount of calcium needed to maintain bone mass. Based on the 1991 *Harvard Health Letter Special Report,* women in their 40s should get 1,000 to 1,500 milligrams of calcium a day. That amount is increased to 1,500 milligrams for women after menopause. Requiring even more calcium, pregnant and breastfeeding women need between 1,500 and 2,000 milligrams a day. Because your body can absorb only about 600 milligrams of calcium at a time, it is advisable to take your supplements in two doses, preferably with breakfast and dinner.

Given the statistics, there is an excellent chance you fall into the 75 percent of women who are not getting the calcium they need to stay even, especially if you do not consume large amounts of milk and dairy products. The solution is simple and inexpensive: Either change your diet to include enough calcium-rich foods to make up the difference or take a calcium supplement (see Chapter 6, "Nutrition and Exercise").

All calcium supplements are not created equal. Because calcium comes in many different forms and levels of quality, it is important to make sure you get what you pay for. To be properly absorbed, calcium supplements must dissolve quickly in the stomach. Test your tablets by dropping one into a container filled with 2 to 4 ounces of vinegar and give it a stir every now and then. After thirty minutes, it should be completely dissolved. If not, change brands or look for a different type of calcium supplement.

When a daily dosage is recommended, it means ingestion of *elemental* calcium. Read the label carefully. If the calcium is not specified as elemental, you will have to do some calculating to determine the amount of actual calcium it contains. Listed below is a conversion chart you can use when shopping for a calcium supplement.

TYPE OF CALCIUM	SIZE OF TABLET (MG)	PERCENTAGE AMOUNT OF ELEMENTAL CALCIUM BY WEIGHT	CONVERTED AMOUNT OF ELEMENTAL CALCIUM (MG)
Calcium carbonate	500	40	200
	750	40	300
Calcium citrate	500	21	105
Calcium gluconate	500	9	45
Calcium lactate	650	13	85

Calcium citrate is the preferred choice of many doctors because it is easily absorbed, especially by older women who make less gastric hydrochloric acid. Calcium carbonate and calcium gluconate are also effective but may cause flatulence and constipation. In general, it is best to avoid calcium sources such as bone meal or dolomite, which may contain lead or other heavy metals. Both chelated calcium and calcium phosphate should be passed over as they may not be absorbed by the body. Hydroxyapatite is high in phosphorus and is not as efficiently absorbed as calcium citrate or calcium carbonate.

Antacids are an entirely different issue. Popping antacids has become epidemic in the United States, and manufacturers have lost no time in jumping on the osteoporosis bandwagon to promote yet another feature of this medication. With alternatives like calcium-rich food and pure calcium supplements, it is questionable why anyone would look to an antacid tablet as a primary source of calcium.

To begin with, many antacids contain aluminum, which can actually cause your body to lose calcium; Tums and Titralac are the only readily available nonaluminum antacids. Certain pre-existing medical conditions can also be aggravated by antacids, including colitis, stomach or intestinal bleeding, irregular heart-beat, and kidney disease. They are not recommended for pregnant and breastfeeding women. Finally, taken five to six times a week, antacids can cause constipation and may lead to the formation of kidney stones and other urinary problems.

Although Tums remains an inexpensive source of calcium, it may be worth the effort to look beyond antacids for calcium supplementation.

There seems to be some question among many women as to the effectiveness of taking calcium if you are no longer making significant amounts of estrogen or decide not to take hormone replacement therapy. Yes, estrogen does increase the absorption of calcium into your system. However, even without estrogen, natural or supplemented, your body will absorb calcium but at a lower rate. Scientists have not done enough work in this area to say definitively how much less calcium is absorbed. So, if you are postmenopausal and not on hormone replacement therapy, you may want to increase the recommended daily calcium intake by 20 to 30 percent, but be sure to check with your physician before doing so.

What about vitamin D? Simply put, it is essential in order for your body to absorb calcium. Unfortunately, there are very few foods in our diet rich in vitamin D. Most people manage to get some vitamin D by consuming milk, bread, cereal, or foods to which it has been added. Exposure to sunshine can also trigger the formation of vitamin D, but because of varying conditions like rainy days, the use of sunscreens and makeup, the amount of skin exposed to the sun, and length of exposure, this method of getting vitamin D is not considered reliable. To ensure adequate levels of vitamin D, many physicians prescribe a multivitamin that contains the recommended daily dosage of 400 international units. There is also at least one product on the market that combines 1,200 milligrams of elemental calcium and 400 international units of vitamin D, probably the ideal combination for women from early perimenopause right through postmenopause.

It is important to avoid taking too much vitamin D; more than 1,000 units a day can actually increase bone loss.

Magnesium is another important mineral and is necessary for skeletal health. Although sometimes debated, doctors agree that magnesium dosage should be half of the amount of calcium you take on a daily basis—600 milligrams magnesium to 1,200 milligrams of calcium. Although magnesium deficiency is rare among women who eat a balanced diet, supplementation is necessary in women who are malnourished, anorexic, bulimic, or alcoholic.

Although vitamin K is necessary for blood clotting, it is also important in bone building and repair. Fortunately, because vitamin K is found in many vegetables, deficiency is rare. Nevertheless, low vegetable consumption and frequent use of antibiotics can cause a deficiency and increase your risk for osteoporosis. Proper diet will usually solve the problem.

Some quick reminders about vitamin and mineral supplements:

- Do not take more than the recommended daily dosage: more is not better and in some cases can be extremely harmful.
- Take calcium supplements and vitamin D at mealtimes or just before you go to bed; they are absorbed into the system more efficiently at that time.
- If you take a calcium supplement, be sure to take vitamin D; without it, the calcium you take will not be absorbed.

Evaluate Estrogen Replacement. It is difficult to read a newspaper or magazine these days without seeing an article on hormone replacement therapy. One of the most controversial topics in medicine today, this issue is discussed in depth in the next chapter. However, one of the clear benefits of estrogen replacement is its proven ability to prevent or delay the effects of osteoporosis.

One of only two drugs approved by the Food and Drug Administration (FDA) for the treatment of osteoporosis, estrogen has been found to have a positive effect on bone formation. Specifically, long-term estrogen replacement therapy has been proven to prevent osteoporosis in 75 to 80 percent of women. It is especially effective in women with chemically or surgically induced menopause, who have had an abrupt loss of estrogen production. The effectiveness of estrogen replacement seems to center around its immediate use after the onset of menopause and its continuation for eight to ten years, the time when women experience bone loss at an accelerated rate. After that, when therapy is discontinued, bone loss does resume but at a much slower rate, usually associated with the normal effects of aging.

Estrogen has also been shown to have a positive effect during perimenopause and even many years after the onset of menopause. Dr. Bockman says, "During the perimenopausal period, for women who are estrogen deficient, estrogen replacement is beneficial and may even augment bone mass. It has a direct effect on those cells that are responsible for making bone, a fact that was not known until two or three years ago. New data are coming out that indicate estrogen may also be beneficial later in life, not just during the rapid bone loss period immediately following menopause."

If you are sold on the idea of taking hormone replacement therapy as a deterrent to osteoporosis, it is important to be sure that your calcium, vitamin D, and magnesium intake are at the recommended levels in order for replacement therapy to be fully effective.

All of this probably sounds like just the ticket, but there are still many unknowns about estrogen replacement and osteoporosis. For example, how long should the therapy last and how strong does the dosage need to be? Should replacement therapy be administered for only twenty-five days a month or on a continuous basis every day? Is estrogen replacement delivered via a patch as effective as tablets? Take some time to carefully read Chapter 4, "Hormone Replacement Therapy." Many of your questions will be answered and you will have the information you need to make a better decision about estrogen replacement and osteoporosis.

Examine Calcitonin. Besides estrogen, the hormone calcitonin is the only drug approved by the FDA for the treatment of osteoporosis. Calcitonin is secreted by the thyroid gland and helps inhibit bone loss. It has only recently been used as a drug in the treatment of women who already have osteoporosis and the results, although positive, have not been tested over a significant period of time. Current testing is focused on the use of calcitonin as a preventive for osteoporosis and is in the preliminary stages of investigation.

Although the side effects are mild, the down side of calcitonin is that it is expensive and can only be taken by injection in the United States, as opposed to in Europe, where it is administered as a nasal spray. Researchers in the United States are now studying the effectiveness of calcitonin as a nasal spray in the prevention of bone loss during the early postmenopausal years.

Experimental Drugs

Not yet approved by the FDA, other drugs, such as etidronate, thiazides, fluoride, calcitriol, and parathyroid hormone, are still in the testing phase for their effectiveness in the prevention and treatment of osteoporosis. Each of these drugs has had some promising results, but testing is still in the experimental stages, and it will be many years before we know with certainty what works.

As frustrating as this may seem, there is often good reason for delayed approval by the FDA. Many of us hear only about the good results of tests and think the FDA is holding out on us. Yet in some cases, the entire picture has not been provided by the media or even the researchers. Katie Maslow, senior analyst at the U.S. Congress Office of Technology Assessment, offers this salient example: "In the case of etidronate, the *New England Journal of Medicine* published two articles in the spring and summer of 1990 that talked about increased bone mass and decreased fracture. Very quickly after that, the results of the third year of study of etidronate showed more fractures in the treatment group than in the nontreatment group. Consequently, the FDA has withheld approval of the drug, waiting for the fourth- and fifth-year data, which will be published shortly. In the interim, the drug is available, women hear about it, doctors have limited information, none know about the existence of additional information, and the drug may be prescribed without all the facts being known."

It is important to pay attention to the rulings of the FDA. Taking a drug that is not approved for a specific condition is risky, and this is one time, in particular, when you should understand that what you hear on the news may not be the final story.

The Future

Because more than 20 million people in the United States are affected at an annual cost exceeding $10 billion, osteoporosis is a very hot subject. The good news is that there is an enormous amount of research being conducted on issues such as

- Identification of new risk factors and further study of existing ones.
- Improved methods for measurement of bone mass.
- The relationship of calcium intake to bone loss.
- Identification of which age groups most benefit from the effects of exercise.
- Increased understanding of the mechanism of estrogen and progesterone action on bone remodeling and mineral metabolism.
- Examination of therapeutic approaches including sodium fluoride, calcitonin, vitamin D metabolites, low-dose parathyroid hormone, bisphosphonates, and anabolic steroids.

Unfortunately, the results of this research may occur too late to be useful during our lifetime. So we will all have to work a little harder, perhaps get involved with the National Osteoporosis Foundation (see Appendix 2, "Resources"), accept the fact that there is no miracle cure, and learn about all the options in order to come up with the best action plan possible.

Heart Disease

> The trouble with heart disease is that the first symptom is often hard to deal with: sudden death.
>
> —Michael Phelps, M.D.,
> BBC World Service

We all grew up thinking heart attacks happened only to men. The stereotype was a cigar-smoking, slightly overweight, hard-driving man who dropped dead in his early 50s. Today, that picture has changed. Women are just as likely to die from heart disease as are men. For example, in 1988, of the 509,592 people who died from a heart attack in the United States, almost half of them, 245,087, were women.

Women dying from heart disease is not a new trend. What is new is the attention being paid to health issues of women, especially as they differ from those of men. Up until recently, the majority of research on heart disease centered only on men. However, a woman's body is not like a man's, and it responds differently to disease and sometimes treatment. Heart disease is a prime example. Add the fact that it is the number one cause of death in women, and you have a compelling reason for the new surge in research on women and heart disease.

Sexual Differences

Remember that old schoolyard taunt, "Boys may be bigger, but girls are better." Well, when it comes to risk associated with heart disease, a woman's body really is the preferred model up to a point. The female heart is slightly smaller than a man's, but it is just as strong and has the ability to beat much longer, usually an average of eight years longer. Women also tend to carry fat differently than men, generally in the lower body, like the buttocks and thighs. Upper-body fat, the kind that conjures up pictures of a potbellied stove, is more commonly seen in men and has a direct relationship to heart disease. Moreover, up until the age of 60, women are half as likely to have a heart attack.

Then the picture changes. About ten years after menopause,

women become as vulnerable to heart disease as men. The pendulum swings even farther, and postmenopausal women end up on the wrong end. They have twice the chance of men of developing heart failure after a heart attack and are much less likely to survive hospitalization or a year of recovery. Once they have heart disease, women do not seem to respond as well as men to certain treatments, such as bypass surgery. Women also have a higher incidence of diabetes, a major risk factor, and, after a heart attack, have twice the risk of dying as men with diabetes.

Although we know menopause and the lack of estrogen is a significant risk factor in heart disease, it is still not clear whether postmenopausal women incur additional risk because their symptoms are not recognized in the early stages. Physicians do not perceive women as heart disease candidates, as they do men. Because they are less likely to recommend surgery for women, the disease is often worse by the time they finally schedule it. Consequently, women candidates for heart surgery tend to be older and have smaller coronary arteries than do men, all of which impacts on survival. Physician reluctance to schedule procedures or surgery might also stem from the lack of research in this area and knowledge of female survival rates. What is more, women seem to be less responsive than men when treated with the same anticlotting drug often administered to heart attack patients.

This may mean that the health of your heart is in your hands. Become educated so that you can take an active role in your medical care.

The Facts

Cardiovascular disease is a broad term used to describe a variety of unhealthy conditions related to the heart and blood vessels. These include coronary heart disease, heart attack, stroke, and angina pectoris (extreme chest pain). The most well known of these conditions is heart attack, and although it may cause death, it is actually the result of heart disease, which has probably existed for several years before the fatal occurrence. If you are lucky, you may experience some warning indicators, but more likely, you will need to understand the signs of heart disease, be vigilant about your health, and insist on getting the attention you need from a physician to avoid becoming a statistic.

Heart disease in any form relates to the ability of blood to flow uninterrupted to the heart. When blood flow is decreased or partially blocked, it puts stress on the heart and, depending on the severity, may eventually lead to a heart attack or impairment of other vital organs.

Excess cholesterol is the culprit in reduced blood flow. Made up of fatty material, *cholesterol* is a waxy substance produced by the liver. In most cases, the liver is able to manufacture all the cholesterol you require. Therefore, when you eat foods high in cholesterol, you provide more than your body needs. Basically, the extra cholesterol remains in the bloodstream and forms globules, better known as *plaque*, which attach to the walls of the arteries. This condition is called *atherosclerosis* and is the most common form of heart disease. Once attached, the plaque usually stays put, narrowing the artery and making your heart pump that much harder just to keep the blood flow going. Sometimes, the plaque breaks off from the artery walls, forms a clot, and can partially or completely block the artery and cause an embolism. No blood flow, no nourishment of vital organs, not a good situation.

The Statistics

Although you probably have a relative or know someone who suffered a heart attack, you might still find it difficult to appreciate your potential risk for heart disease. Here are some sobering statistics:

- One out of every three women 65 years and older has some form of heart disease.
- Out of 2,000 postmenopausal women in a single year, 20 will get heart disease and 12 will die from it.
- There is a greater risk of dying from heart disease than from cancer. Women die from heart disease at a rate of two to one over all forms of cancer and ten to one over breast cancer.

- The death rate from heart disease and stroke is significantly higher for black women than for white: a 19 percent higher rate from heart disease and a 79 percent higher death rate from stroke.

Risk Factors

In many ways, heart disease is not a complex issue from the patient standpoint. Sufficient research has been done with both men and women to identify the risk factors most likely to cause heart disease. Moreover, the majority of them can be controlled by you. But these risk factors must be taken seriously. Do not skim the list, decide only a few apply, and feel that you are off the hook. The more risk factors you have, the greater your chance of developing heart disease. For example, if you smoke and have high blood pressure and an elevated cholesterol level, your risk of heart disease can be eight times greater than that of someone who has only one risk factor.

Family History. Your greatest risk of having heart disease, and one that you cannot do anything about, comes down to the gene pool. If someone in your immediate family suffered from heart disease, especially before the age of 60, you are much more likely to develop the disease. Just because you did not know your grandfather or never got along with your older sister, you should not ignore the facts. If either of them died from a heart attack or suffered a stroke, you are a likely candidate for heart disease.

High Blood Cholesterol. Women used to brag about their measurements, accomplishments at work, or latest vacation. Today, they flaunt their cholesterol levels, often without understanding what they really mean. All sorts of numbers and terms get thrown around randomly: "My LDL is way down." "I lowered my overall cholesterol count to under 200." "My count is 245, but because my HDL is so high, my doctor says I don't have to worry." Half of us go around feeling smug, and the rest worry about what the next tests will look like.

We all know having a high cholesterol count is hazardous to

our health, but very few of us know how to look at the numbers and make sense of them. Here are some quick definitions:

- *High-density lipoproteins* (HDL) transport excess cholesterol in the blood to the liver for excretion. Also known as the "good cholesterol" in measuring blood cholesterol, high levels of HDL create a protective effect against heart disease.
- *Low-density lipoproteins* (LDL), or "bad cholesterol," store cholesterol in the blood. Because the liver makes most of the required cholesterol, the excess stored in the LDL remains in the bloodstream and eventually attaches itself to artery walls and causes atherosclerosis.

To get to the heart of the cholesterol count issue, you need to have a meaningful measurement that separates the good (HDL) from the bad (LDL). Obviously a combined number can easily distort the picture. One of the easiest and most consistent ways to measure your cholesterol is to examine the percentage of good cholesterol (HDL) to your overall cholesterol count, which includes both good and bad cholesterol. For example, if your HDL is 45 and your overall cholesterol count is 200, your proportion of HDL is about 23 percent ($45 \div 200 = 0.225$, or 23 percent).

Now to determine your risk for heart disease based on your percentage of good cholesterol, look at the following table.

Risk of Developing Heart Disease

PERCENTAGE OF HDL/ CHOLESTEROL	LEVEL OF RISK
28 or higher	Very little
23–28	Below average
18–22	Average
9–17	High
Less than 9	Dangerous

Source: Penny Wise Budoff, *No More Hot Flashes* (New York: Warner Books, 1984), p. 286.

Many physicians and laboratories use another method of calculating the risk of coronary heart disease by using a figure that represents your cholesterol/HDL ratio. Using the previous example, this ratio can be calculated by dividing your total cholesterol by your HDL ($200 \div 45 = 4.4$).

RATIO OF CHOLESTEROL/HDL	LEVEL OF RISK
Less than 3.5	Protection probable
3.5 to 4.4	Below average
4.5 to 5.5	Average
5.6 to 10.9	High
11 or greater	Dangerous

Source: Penny Wise Budoff, *No More Hot Flashes* (New York: Warner Books, 1984), p. 286.

Take these numbers seriously and be honest with yourself about your risk level.

Menopause. A factor obviously out of your control, reaching menopause significantly increases your risk of developing heart disease. Up until that time, women are usually protected from heart disease by estrogen, which automatically keeps cholesterol levels in check. After menopause, it is a whole new ball game. For reasons still not completely understood, lack of estrogen causes the ratio of good cholesterol to bad cholesterol to shift dramatically, usually within six months after menopause. This results in an increased overall cholesterol level for the postmenopausal woman but, more significantly, a level that has a higher proportion of bad cholesterol. Although this shift is most dramatic after menopause, changes in cholesterol can often be detected during perimenopause. Ask your doctor to monitor your cholesterol annually from the age of 40.

Menopause is the risk factor, not age. Women with early menopause, whether it occurs naturally or as a result of surgery, have twice the risk of developing heart disease as women of the same age who have not had menopause.

High Blood Pressure (Hypertension). Known as the silent killer, high blood pressure and its symptoms are usually not readily apparent. An explosive temper or type A personality is not necessarily an indicator of the condition. Hypertension is quite common. Half of all women over 55 have high blood pressure, and it seems to be more prevalent and severe among black women. Unless you have your blood pressure checked regularly, a painless and quick procedure, you may not know you have the condition until it has already done some damage.

Blood pressure refers to the amount of force put on the walls of the arteries as blood is pumped throughout your body. The measurement includes two numbers: The first, systolic pressure, indicates the pressure as your heart beats; the second, diastolic, is the pressure that remains in your arteries between heartbeats. The pressure fluctuates throughout the day depending on what you are doing. Normal blood pressure is 120/80, and most physicians concentrate on the second number. If your diastolic pressure is 90 or higher, you should definitely consult your doctor.

High blood pressure exists only when it consistently remains above normal levels and is a sign of heart disease. For example, if your arteries are narrowed because of excess cholesterol and you have atherosclerosis, your heart will have to pump harder to push the blood through. Low blood pressure means less of a chance of developing other conditions that put additional strain on your heart, such as heart attack, stroke, and kidney disease.

Smoking. Clear the air—smoking does absolutely nothing beneficial for your body. In fact, it is disastrous for your health, especially after menopause. When it comes to heart disease, smoking damages the blood vessel walls and makes them easy targets for plaque buildup. This turns you into a prime candidate for atherosclerosis. That means:

- Smoking causes more deaths from heart disease than from cancer.
- Smoking accounts for 41 percent of coronary deaths among women.

- Smokers have a two to four times greater risk of sudden cardiac death than nonsmokers.
- Smoking has been linked strongly to a higher incidence of stroke.
- Women who smoke are two to six times as likely to suffer a heart attack as nonsmokers.
- Women who smoke tend to have menopause earlier, thus increasing the risk of heart disease.
- Female smokers who also take birth control pills are up to thirty-nine times more likely to have a heart attack and up to twenty-two times more likely to have a stroke than nonsmokers who do not use oral contraceptives.
- Smoking increases the relative risk of dying from heart disease by 70 percent.

Scary stuff? You bet, and enough to motivate you to quit. Within two to three years of quitting, a smoker's chance of suffering a heart attack drops to the level of a lifelong non-smoker. This is one heart disease risk factor you can do something about.

Diabetes. Often called a woman's disease, twice as many women as men develop diabetes after age 45. Diabetes, also known as *high blood sugar,* is a serious risk factor and doubles your risk of death from heart disease.

Diabetes and being overweight go hand in hand—more than 85 percent of all diabetics are at least 20 percent overweight. Additional risk factors for diabetes include family history of the condition, being Jewish or nonwhite, and living below the poverty level.

Overweight. Nag, nag, nag. You have heard it all before, but perhaps the combination of being overweight and the risk of developing heart disease will grab your attention. Although extra weight might limit hot flashes for some because of the estrogen stored in fat cells, those extra pounds still do more harm than good. Overweight by how much, you ask? Some doctors say in excess of 30 percent of your ideal weight. Others feel 15 extra pounds or more is too much.

What is your ideal weight supposed to be? This is not an easy call, given the weight tables available today. For example, the popular Metropolitan Life Insurance Weight Table (1983) is not only out-of-date, but also out of sync with current thinking on body weight and long-term good health. Based on mortality statistics more than ten years old, the life insurance tables do not break down recommended weight by age, nor do they account for the fact that muscle tissue weighs more than fat. Using these kinds of tables, many athletes would be considered overweight because of their high percentage of muscle to fat.

Weight is obviously not the whole picture. A better way to determine if you weigh too much is to measure how much fat your body has in proportion to lean body tissue composed of muscle, bone, water, salt, and everything else besides fat. Commonly known as *body fat measurement,* this calculation can determine how physically fit you really are. Which of these two women of similar height and body frame is in better shape for long-term good health: the one who weighs 115 and never exercises or the other who works out regularly and weighs in at 123?

Body fat measurement is not an exact science, but the three methods for determining percentage of body fat—underwater weighing, skinfold measurement, and electrical impedance testing—are accurate enough to help you monitor your eating and exercise habits. Many variables can distort results, such as your menstrual cycle if you tend to retain water just before menstruating, but overall, it is a more effective way to measure fitness than by scale weight. Testing should be performed by a trained and experienced professional, either in your doctor's office, hospital, reputable health club, or YWCA.

As a footnote, the average college female has 25 percent body fat while the average middle-aged woman has 32 percent body fat, with the healthy range for midlife women varying between 20 and 30 percent. You are at increased risk for heart disease, diabetes, and stroke if your body fat percentage exceeds 33. This is not the time to split hairs—you know if you are overweight. Take a hard look at the potential damage this can do to your body.

Women who are overweight have a much higher chance of developing heart disease even if they have no other risk factors. Being 20 percent or more above the desirable weight can double your risk of heart disease. The irony is that most overweight people do have other risk factors such as high blood pressure, high cholesterol, and diabetes. There is no health benefit to being overweight, and most of the time it is extremely harmful. Arriving at and maintaining an ideal weight is a battle but one worth fighting to maintain good health.

Your Options

In order to avoid losing up to thirty years of good healthy living after menopause, you are going to have to do a few things to protect your body from heart disease. Listed below are several options to consider. However, doing nothing is not one of them. Wake up and be proactive.

Recognize Symptoms and Risk Factors and See Your Doctor. As a child, I remember peeking at medical books belonging to my best friend's father and being scared out of my wits by pictures of dread diseases and bizarre abnormalities. When I grew up and perused medical guides written for nondoctors, I was just as terrified by reading lists of symptoms of various diseases—certain that I either already had the symptoms or, by knowing about them, would be sure to develop the disease. I honestly believed that if I remained ignorant of the symptoms, I would never develop the affliction.

Silly as this may sound, many people feel the same way. Well, this is not the time to put your head in the sand. You will not get heart disease just by knowing the warning signs. Nor will you turn into a hypochondriac, imagining you have all the symptoms and suddenly having a heart attack.

Remember, because the symptoms usually appear in the form of a heart attack, most people do not realize they have heart disease until it is well advanced. Therefore, it is important to know and pay attention to the early warning signs and risk factors associated with the disease:

- Chest pain, also known as angina, is usually the precursor of a heart attack. This does not mean a single brief, sharp pain across your chest occurring every now and then. Angina is spasmodic, choking, or suffocating chest pain that usually disappears with rest but continues to occur on a regular basis.
- High blood pressure.
- High blood cholesterol level.
- Being overweight.
- Smoking.
- Sedentary lifestyle.
- Diabetes.

Now that you are aware of the symptoms and risk factors, go see your doctor and specifically discuss them as they relate to your risk for heart disease. Many physicians are less aggressive in treating women as potential heart disease patients than men. Believe it or not, you may have to take the initiative. It is not enough for you just to accept your doctor's advice and try to lower your blood pressure or cholesterol. Ask questions about heart disease, your risk, and methods of treatment. Make sure all the cards are on the table and you walk away feeling confident and in control. If you blow it and forget to ask a question or two or even lose your nerve, make another appointment and get the answers.

Change Your Eating Habits Forever. Face it, you have probably tried various diets over the years with minimal success. Most diets are setups for failure and leave you feeling down about yourself. People use diets as temporary regimens to get back into shape. If and when they succeed, they often revert to bad habits and regain the weight they lost.

Keeping your weight down is not a natural act. It is something you need to work on all the time, including weekends and holidays. I know how hard it can be because I was overweight as a child. By the time I was in seventh grade, my mother had had enough of my overeating. She threw out all the candy and cookies in the house and forced me to lose weight by eating properly. Her threats about turning into a circus fat lady if I ate an ice-cream cone were a little heavy-handed, but in the end, they did the trick. Because I still love to eat and gain weight easily, I watch my weight like a hawk and with exercise am able to enjoy food without guilt and extra pounds.

Once you lose the extra pounds and figure out how to maintain your weight, you will be able to put the energy you wasted worrying about being overweight to much better use. Imagine the sense of freedom of not having to obsess about your weight and the extra time you will have for the activities you really enjoy.

View this as an opportunity to kill two birds with one stone—overweight and high blood cholesterol.

I wear a size 8, which is pretty thin, but it's been a lot of work to get here. Fifteen years ago I was into the real yo-yo diet routine. I'd go up to 150, come down to 130, back up again to 160, and down to 140. In fact, I was up and down most of my life, but now manage to stay around 123 to 125. The difference for me was getting involved with Overeaters Anonymous, a group that has a twelve-step program and meets a few times a week. Even though I'm relatively thin now, I don't think I could stay this way without some constant support. It's so easy to get caught up in thinking about food all the time. . . . What am I going to eat for dinner, or how am I going to diet today? All that chatter in your head takes away from thinking about anything else that's going on in your life. I'm much freer now that I no longer have to deal with being overweight.

Married mother, 59

So, how do you get to this ideal position and keep heart disease at bay? Start by eliminating the word *diet*, which usually describes a temporary way of eating. Take the first step and eliminate it from your vocabulary once and for all. It just does not apply to what you must do to maintain a healthy body. What we are talking about is a lifetime commitment.

The second step is to think about a permanent change in the way you approach eating. As an adult, you should know what foods to eat and what to avoid. For a quick review, take a look at Chapter 6, "Nutrition and Exercise." Like the federal government, your eating habits should be a series of checks and balances. If you avoid desserts all week, you should feel guilt-less about enjoying an ice-cream sundae over the weekend. Be realistic about the food you put into your body. Plan what you eat so that you give yourself "time off" and indulge in treats once in a while. Understand your limits. To maintain your weight, it is probably more realistic to assume only one or two meals a week of wild and crazy eating, with no snacking between meals.

Depending on your degree of commitment, the third step could put you out of the running as a candidate for heart disease. Although the American Heart Association recommends a diet not to exceed 30 percent fat in relation to total food intake per day, a physician in California has done some exciting work that challenges this advice. Using an approach based solely on diet and exercise, as opposed to medication and surgery, Dr. Dean Ornish worked with a group of forty-one men and women with heart disease to determine whether this noninvasive strategy could halt and perhaps reverse the progress of the disease. Half the group received standard cardiac care, with no change in their diet or exercise regimen. The other half, Dr. Ornish's group, were put on a rigorous vegetarian diet with no more than 10 percent of the calories coming from fat. They also engaged in moderate exercise, about a half-hour walk each day; practiced stress management for an hour, including yoga, meditation, and breathing exercises; and stopped smoking.

The results were astonishing even after the first year:

	DR. ORNISH'S GROUP	STANDARD CARDIAC CARE GROUP
Arterial blockages	Reduced in 82% of the group	Increased in the majority of cases
Chest pain	Reduced by 91%	Increased by 165%

Becoming a vegetarian and eating an extremely low-fat diet may seem radical to you at the moment, but after working with patients with heart disease, Dr. Ornish has a different outlook: "I don't understand why asking people to eat a well-balanced vegetarian diet is considered drastic while it is medically conservative to cut people open or put them on powerful cholesterol-lowering drugs the rest of their lives."

You may not subscribe to Dr. Ornish's philosophy, but it is difficult to ignore the results he achieved with diet and exercise. Translated, it is clear that improving on the recommendation of the American Heart Association can only benefit you. Give it a try, a little at a time, and do it in a way that allows you to succeed.

Slowly, over the past few years, I have become more and more of a vegetarian. I don't eat red meat and seldom eat chicken and fish anymore. The last time I went to my holistic doctor for a checkup, he was thrilled with my blood tests. My calcium level was higher, and my cholesterol was the lowest it's ever been.

Single woman, 54

Get the Lead Out and Exercise. By the time you reached 35, it might have occurred to you that exercise was not a natural part of your daily routine. Maybe you no longer had toddlers to carry everywhere or perhaps your full-time job did not have an exercise recess in the afternoon. Your figure was still in pretty good shape, however, and you probably assumed you could beat the odds and keep your fit appearance effortlessly.

What a surprise when you turned 40, looked around, and noticed that some parts of your body had migrated from their original location. If you did nothing to rectify the situation then, by the time you reached 50, you probably suffered from lack of energy; flabbiness in your upper arms, stomach, buttocks, and thighs; and some unwanted pounds on top of everything else. Moreover, you now faced a new potential threat to your body—heart disease.

Although regular, vigorous exercise will not cure all that ails you, it is incredibly beneficial and will help you

- Lose extra pounds.
- Control your blood pressure.
- Increase the level of good cholesterol (HDL).
- Prevent diabetes.
- Condition your lungs.
- Tone muscles.
- Keep joints supple.
- Maintain bone density levels.
- Build stamina.
- Manage stress.

Time is up. You can no longer turn your back on exercise; it is a required part of good healthy living and will make a significant difference in the length and quality of your life. The key to making exercise work for you is to set yourself up to succeed. This means choosing an activity that is relatively easy to do, fits your schedule, and is one that you enjoy. You must exercise regularly, at least thirty minutes every day or sixty minutes three times a week, to gain any benefit (see Chapter 6, "Nutrition and Exercise").

Some women are fortunate to have older women as role models. Look around and you may be able to spot the kind of active woman mentioned below.

I think I'm going to get better looking as I get older. I don't mean in terms of physical beauty, I'm talking about aging well. Unless something happens to me physically and I'm unable to exercise, I plan to keep my body in excellent condition. I love seeing older women with gray hair jogging, out walking, or being very active. One of my friends I play tennis with is in her late 50s. She goes to two exercise classes every morning, plays tennis four days a week, and is on a weight program for muscle strengthening. She is in amazing physical condition and is a marvel to me. I mean she doesn't have "grandma arms" or a big stomach. She just takes great care of herself.

Married woman, 45

Consider the Estrogen Option. Because estrogen raises the good cholesterol (HDL) levels in the blood, it is often considered a potential weapon in the fight against heart disease. Nevertheless, estrogen replacement has always been a controversial subject. It seems that a day does not pass without a new article appearing on the pros and cons of estrogen therapy. Some doctors advocate it as the elixir for the middle-aged woman, whereas others attack it as an untested drug with potentially life-threatening consequences. Still other physicians recommend its limited use in the prevention of osteoporosis and, until recently, heart disease.

This woman uses hormone replacement therapy as part of a total program to prevent heart disease.

There's no way I'm going to die of a heart attack, especially with all of the help out there that's available. My cholesterol level was always modestly elevated until I started taking hormones. Ideally, I would like to take as little estrogen as possible and still get some protection for my heart, given that I plan to take it for the rest of my life. But I also cut out almost all the fat in my diet. I use exercise as another weapon and feel very much in control.

Married mother, 49

The picture, however, is not completely rosy. Although the data are fairly clear on the benefits of using estrogen replacement as a preventive for osteoporosis, they are less clear for heart disease. Studies done to date show significant positive effects, but the research methods used cast doubt on the results. Here are some of the reasons why:

- The majority of tests on the effects of estrogen therapy and heart disease have not been randomized. This means that there was not a mixture of women in varying degrees of health from different economic and ethnic backgrounds. Furthermore, the subjects were able to choose whether or not they wanted estrogen treatment.

- Women who take estrogen after menopause are more likely to be white, educated, upper middle class, and in good health, thereby at lower risk of heart disease than women who do not. These are the populations that have been studied to date.
- In a ten-year Nurses' Health Study involving 49,000 post-menopausal women, results published in the *New England Journal of Medicine* in September 1991 indicated the risk of heart disease was 44 percent lower among women who took estrogen than among those who did not. However, this study was not randomized, and many of the women not on estrogen were obese and physically inactive, thus putting them at greater risk for heart disease. All of this adds up to uncertainty about the existing test results.

Then there is the issue of drug administration. Women without a uterus have the advantage of being able to take estrogen by itself, also referred to as *unopposed estrogen*. Because of the risk of uterine cancer when estrogen is unopposed, however, women with a uterus who elect to take estrogen must also take progesterone. So what is the big deal? Unfortunately, progesterone has been shown to significantly lessen the positive effect of estrogen on blood cholesterol levels.

What is a woman to do? You can wait it out and hope that new test results will be more precise. Or you can opt for hormone replacement therapy and keep an eye on the latest research as results are published. Either way, it will be to your benefit to spend more time learning about hormone replacement therapy as discussed in Chapter 4.

Assess Aspirin as a Preventive. A landmark study completed a few years ago demonstrated that a single aspirin taken once a day was effective in reducing the risk of heart attack in men. Aspirin, which inhibits blood clotting, was shown to prevent heart attacks by keeping clots from forming and possibly blocking a coronary artery.

In 1991, data from the Nurses' Health Study indicated that heart attack risk was also reduced by 25 percent in women who took one to six aspirins per week; the benefit was especially prominent in women over 50. The problem is, the Nurses' Health Study was not set up to evaluate the use of aspirin. Consequently, nurses took aspirin as needed to relieve headaches and not as part of a regimented program. The jury is still out on this one, but a long-term study on women like the one done on men is in the works. However, the results will not be available for at least five years.

Be careful. Although aspirin is considered to be a safe drug, taking one a day over many years will expose you to possible serious side effects like intestinal bleeding. For now, talk to your doctor about the latest information on this subject before taking aspirin on a regular basis to prevent heart attacks.

One Clear Thought. Yes, it is confusing. To put things in perspective, take a moment to reflect on the following statistic raised at an FDA hearing on estrogen and heart disease:

> Without the use of drugs, heart disease in women could be reduced by 90 percent if women would increase their exercise, lose weight, eat less fat, monitor blood pressure, and stop smoking.

The Future

A great deal of research still needs to be done on women and heart disease. Simply put, the medical community has realized the error of its ways in excluding women from previous heart disease research and is trying to make up for lost time. Although this will entail an enormous effort at high cost, the results will be invaluable in saving many thousands of lives each year. Until the results are in, you will have to make sure your complaints are heard and work closely with your physician, understanding you will be treated as if no gender difference exists.

Listed below is a sampling of some of the research currently in progress or under consideration:

- The three-year PEPI (postmenopausal estrogen/progestin intervention trial) launched in 1991 is the most publicized study on women and heart disease. Administered by the National Heart, Lung and Blood Institute with the collaboration of four other entities of the National Institutes of Health,

  - It involves 840 healthy postmenopausal women, age 45 to 64.
  - It is designed as a randomized double-blind study (neither the doctors nor the patients will know which drug or nondrug they take) testing the effects of estrogen, three different kinds of combined estrogen and progestin, and a placebo (a "fake" pill containing no medication).
  - It will evaluate the effects of estrogen replacement versus a placebo on the following heart disease risk factors: good cholesterol (HDL), blood pressure, fibrinogen (blood factor predictor), and insulin.

Although comprehensive in scope, this study will not measure the occurrence of heart attacks and other cardiac symptoms. Two other follow-up studies are being considered: a prevention trial to determine whether hormone replacement therapy reduces the incidence of heart disease in healthy women and a trial of women who already have heart disease to determine whether hormone replacement therapy reduces the incidence of heart attack.

- The National Institutes of Health is considering a study of 60,000 women to be followed over a ten-year period, testing hormone, diet, and lifestyle intervention in the prevention of heart disease.
- Also sponsored by the National Institutes of Health is a

study on the long-term effects of aspirin as a preventive for heart disease. Similar to a previous study on men, it will involve 40,000 postmenopausal female nurses. It will also evaluate the effects of β-carotene and vitamin E on women's risk for heart disease.

Wrinkles

Everyone gets wrinkles sooner or later. Contrary to popular belief, they do not suddenly occur as soon as you become postmenopausal. Menopause does not cause wrinkles, but decreasing amounts of estrogen contribute to thinning skin. Be honest: You noticed skin changes in your early 40s, probably before you even gave a single thought to menopause. In fact, studies have shown that most women in their 30s and 40s fear wrinkles more than they do any other part of being old.

However, wrinkles are a part of life, and everyone seems to cope with them differently. This woman's attitude was probably influenced by her lack of wrinkles so far. It will be interesting to see how her thinking changes as time goes by.

I happen to come from a family that has good genes and can get away with wearing very little makeup. I'm lucky—I don't have that many wrinkles. Plastic surgery isn't something I would consider right now. Maybe in ten years, but not now. I have friends who've had their busts lifted and tummies tucked. But I don't feel I need it. I'm very secure in what my body is like and what it can do.

Married mother, 48

How Wrinkles Happen

You have heard it before, so this should come as no surprise: Sun damage causes 80 percent of all wrinkles. Stop for a minute and let this fact sink in. If you stayed out of the sun as a child and wore serious sunscreen protection when exposed, you would probably have the skin of a 20-year-old. There is no mystery about what causes the majority of wrinkles, but for some reason most people ignore the facts and continue to offer up their skin to the sun's damaging rays.

Most of the remaining 20 percent of wrinkles are related to your personality. You laugh, you cry, you get angry, you smile, and what do you get? Wrinkles. Every time you use your facial muscles to express yourself you use up some of the natural elasticity of your skin. Over time, this elasticity starts to give out just like an overused rubber band.

Abrasive soaps and cosmetics and natural thinning of the skin that comes with aging also contribute to wrinkles. As your estrogen supply decreases, the fatty layer below the surface, which supports the skin and makes it look plump and youthful, starts to disappear. Without this fatty layer, already damaged and wrinkled skin will become more noticeable. Remember, most of your wrinkles will still be a result of unprotected exposure to the sun.

No one is exempt from wrinkles, but the timing and severity depend on genetics, personality, and skin care. Blacks seem to have a ten-year advantage over white women because they start out with thicker skin and darker pigment, which helps protect them from the sun. Still, they end up just as wrinkled as whites. Darker-skinned Caucasians with Mediterranean lineage do better than fair-skinned women with northern European backgrounds. However, dark skin will still not protect you from sun damage. Women who spent summers working on the ultimate tan will wrinkle sooner than those who religiously used sunscreen since early childhood. Women with animated personalities and expressive faces will probably beat out their duller, more passive counterparts for having the most wrinkles.

How to Straighten Yourself Out

To date, very little research has been done on wrinkles, mostly because they are considered a cosmetic, not a medical, problem. With more than 40 million women becoming menopausal in the next decade, however, perhaps the drug and cosmetic companies will find it financially advantageous to launch some long-term studies in the next few years. However, the discovery of a real antidote to wrinkles is highly unlikely.

In the interim, no matter how damaged your skin may be, there are still things you can do to prevent it from getting worse. Assuming you have twenty to thirty years left on the planet, there is no reason to look in the mirror, feel depressed about a few wrinkles, and admit defeat. After all, if you do nothing, you can count on twenty to thirty years' worth of additional damage. Make some changes in how you protect your skin today, and you can bet on improvement in the way you will look tomorrow.

Daily Sunscreen. For some reason, this is a difficult concept to get through most women's minds. The sun is out there shining every day, even when it is cloudy. Yet most women apply sunscreen only when they go to the beach or pool and sometimes not even then.

Get with the program. If you want to avoid wrinkles, use sunscreen every day. Rain or shine. Make it a habit, just like you brush your teeth or apply moisturizer. In fact, there is a trend among cosmetics companies to include a sunscreen in many of their facial moisturizing products. The ideal protection is an SPF 30 sunblock applied over every bit of exposed skin. However, most products contain an SPF 15 or 19, either of which will do the job very nicely. The important thing is to use sunscreen religiously. Also try to remember to wear a hat.

Retin-A. Once heralded as the "fountain of youth in a jar," Retin-A is an effective way to repair certain kinds of damaged skin. Although it is approved by the FDA only as an antiacne medication, many dermatologists use it to treat brown spots and wrinkles. Retin-A works by changing the architecture of the skin and is the only product on the market that can make this claim. Continuous use of Retin-A can actually thicken the skin by increasing skin layers and smoothing out the top of the skin. It is available by prescription in a variety of strengths and should only be used with the close supervision of a dermatologist. Like any drug, it has side effects, which include skin irritation and scaling. It must be applied continuously in order to maintain the positive effects, and avoiding sun exposure is mandatory with its use. This means using sunscreen during the day, every day.

Alpha-Hydroxy Acids. Available over the counter, nonprescription substances such as lactic acid and glycolic acid perform similarly to Retin-A without many of the side effects. Although not as dramatic in their results as Retin-A, alpha-hydroxy acids have a mild effect on wrinkled skin.

Vitamins. Although the reasons are not clear, it seems that vitamins A, C, and E are beneficial to the skin. However, there is a problem with taking megadoses of these or any other vitamins. Do not self-medicate. Get some help from your doctor before taking any pills.

Chemical Peels, Dermabrasion, and Cosmetic Surgery. Women respond differently to the natural aging process and using chemical and surgical intervention is a very individual decision. Unfortunately, the youthful image of women, idealized and displayed in all forms of the media, makes that decision even harder. If only we lived in a society that valued older people, the situation would be very different.

Women who opt to surgically eliminate wrinkles or prop up sagging skin need to be highly motivated. The procedures involved in chemical peels, dermabrasion, or cosmetic surgery are uncomfortable and sometimes extremely painful. With today's sophisticated level of dermatology, however, the results are usually excellent. Many women remain on the fence about surgical and chemical treatments, but this undecided woman is still learning everything she can about her options.

I haven't decided what to do about plastic surgery. It will depend on my work situation and how I feel working next to and competing with 30-year-olds. I've thought about having my breasts raised and made smaller, but I'm chicken. I'm afraid I'll be the one person in a million they're going to screw up and put my eyes

down where my nose is. But I haven't closed the door yet. It really
will depend on what falls, how my eyes look, and whether I can
deal with it. I'm definitely going to try to grow old gracefully.
Meanwhile, I have all kinds of names and information just in case.

Married mother, 53

Spend the time to investigate thoroughly your options and find the kind of dermatologist or plastic surgeon who will be responsive to your needs.

Hormone Replacement Therapy

There is some evidence that both estrogen and progesterone benefit skin condition. Hormone replacement therapy will not make your wrinkles disappear, but it may slow down the aging process and restore a glow to your skin. Estrogen is an important element in maintaining well-toned skin, giving it a thickness and glow associated with youth. Progestin, used with estrogen, has also been shown to improve collagen in the skin, an essential component that keeps the skin firm and resistant to wrinkles. Although hormone replacement therapy is not regularly prescribed for aging skin, the ability to improve skin condition is just one of its many benefits (see Chapter 4, "Hormone Replacement Therapy").

Hair Changes

The one thing I've noticed about menopause is that my skin seems
to be wrinkling a lot faster. I noticed a dramatic change in my
mid-40s. Up until I turned 40, I looked much younger than my
age. Now, I still look younger than my contemporaries, but not by
much. I see myself aging and I also see more facial hair. Not a ton,
but more above my lip and maybe one or two stray hairs that are
dark and coarse on the back of my legs. I guess this is the real
thing—aging. But a pair of tweezers and a little bleach does the

trick. I'm not ready to give up looking good just because some extra wrinkles and weird hair growth have come my way.

Single mother, 47

About five years after menopause, some women experience a change in hair growth. Sprouting what looks like a whisker on your face, noticing thicker hair on your arms, or discovering new hair on your abdomen is alarming but not out of the ordinary. You may also find that the hair on your head is getting thinner and less shiny. No, you will not turn into a bearded lady overnight, nor will you lose all your hair. However, you might feel disheartened about these changes and let them get to you unless you understand what is going on.

As the amount of estrogen in your body decreases, other sex hormones called *androgens*, produced by the ovaries and adrenal glands, begin to have a stronger effect on your body. Although both women and men have them, androgens, often referred to as male hormones, affect several body functions, including libido and hair growth (see Chapter 7, "Sex").

Women have two basic kinds of hair: the soft, fine, thinly growing hair that covers most of your body and the wiry, thicker hair that is responsive to sex hormones and appears on your underarms, face, chest, abdomen, and back. With less estrogen, the effect of androgens on this thicker hair is more significant and often makes it darker, thicker, and even more wiry. It may also cause new hair to grow where it is not welcome. This excess hair growth, also known as *hirsutism*, seems to be hereditary and is more prevalent among women of Mediterranean ancestry. However, not all cases of hirsutism are menopause related, and you should check with a physician for a proper diagnosis.

Hair growth is not the end of the world. Hormone replacement therapy usually counteracts this hair growth. Another approach is to try one of several options for eliminating unwanted hair, such as bleaching, waxing, and electrolysis.

The luster and thickness of the hair on your head is also affected by hormones but, in many instances, may also be the result of hair-styling techniques, thyroid problems, or nutrition.

Unless you have female alopecia, or baldness that occurs earlier in life, it is highly unlikely that you will become bald in middle or old age. However, see a dermatologist if your hair loss persists.

This woman's experience with midlife hair loss is not unusual, but her optimistic attitude about the situation is worth noting.

> I guess my greatest concern is turning into an old lady. I've always been youthful looking, but all of a sudden, the skin on my arms is starting to loosen. And my hair is getting thinner. I've always had long, luxurious auburn hair. It's still long, but it's falling out in fistfuls. I guess it's hereditary because I can remember my mother going through the same thing at my age. The cupboards were full of tar shampoo and every other hair remedy you could think of. But she still has her hair, so I guess I'm not going to lose it all. You never know what's going to happen next as you get older. Just in case, I told my kids that when I'm in a nursing home to make sure that they at least pluck the hairs out of my chin!
>
> Single mother, 52

With all the available ways to cope with midlife hair change, there is no reason to let it get you down. Just take care of it.

Chapter Four

Hormone Replacement Therapy

*There is only one thing about which I am certain, and that
is that there is very little about which one can be certain.*
—W. Somerset Maugham

The Estrogen Question

Up until recently I considered myself very lucky to have been
born when I was. From my earliest memories, medical advances
seemed to happen just when I needed them—the Salk polio
vaccine, birth control pills, intrauterine devices, the flu vaccine.
Now my luck has run out. I am about to reach menopause, and
modern medicine has just not kept pace with my growth. Like
you, I now am faced with conflicting opinions on how to deal
with my body during this major physical change. The prime
example is hormone replacement therapy. Although it is widely
available and comes with some attractive benefits, it has also
been associated with some serious side effects. Even more frustrating is the fact that there still remains a great deal of research
to be done on its long-term use.

Whether or not to take hormone replacement therapy is a big
question with no easy answer. Should you try it for a year or two
just to alleviate hot flashes or continue it indefinitely to lessen
the risk of heart disease and osteoporosis? When should you stop?
What about estrogen and its relation to breast cancer? What
other side effects exist? It is not a slam-dunk decision and the

issues surrounding it are still some of the most hotly debated by doctors today.

Typical of many women facing menopause, this woman's uncertainty may sound familiar.

> *I'm a woman who doesn't know what to do about hormones. I read all the literature, ask all the questions, speak to all the doctors, and still can't make up my mind. There's a part of me that says drugs—I don't want to do it. After all, if I was meant to menstruate all my life, I would be doing it naturally, not with drugs. And then another part of me looks at how helpful drugs have been over the years. So I have all the logical input in my head and still haven't done anything about it.*
>
> Single woman, 53

If the experts cannot agree, how are you supposed to figure out what to do? Not easily perhaps, but by being open-minded and arming yourself with as much knowledge as you can get your hands on, you will be in a position to make a good solid decision and do what is right for you.

Menopause Is Not a Disease

Before you learn about the pros and cons of hormone replacement therapy, it is important to understand the viewpoint of a large part of the medical community on menopause in general. Beginning with some of the earliest medical texts, menopause was often described as a disease. As recently as 1966, Robert A. Wilson, author of *Feminine Forever* (New York: M. Evans, 1966), called it a deficiency disease. Today, doctors commonly describe menopause as a state of hormone deficiency.

The problem with this terminology is that it implies that menopause is a disease that requires a cure or, at the very least, medication to make it better. *Deficiency* is an emotionally charged word that makes you assume that something is inappropriately lacking.

It is not. Remember, menopause is a natural part of the aging process that all women experience. It does not automatically necessitate treatment.

Furthermore, some women feel it is important to experience menopause, that it is a natural part of the aging process. This woman, trained as a nurse, felt strongly enough about menopause and its natural effects to decide against taking hormone replacement therapy.

I have finally accepted menopause as a natural phenomenon. Nature has withdrawn your body's estrogen for a reason, and I don't think it's right to interfere. The body is programmed to react in a certain way, and maybe there's a reason we stop producing estrogen. Does it necessarily have to be bad for everybody? I'm not going to take Premarin just to stop the aging process. I'm a nurse and I've seen 80-year-old women in my practice wearing the estrogen patch. I asked them what happens when they take it off. They said they still get hot flashes. Naturally that's bound to happen when you go off estrogen. You are going to go through menopause no matter what age you are. Sure, it might be less than what you would have gone through otherwise. But still, who are you kidding?

Married mother, 50

A Short History

Estrogen has always been controversial. From the first time it appeared in the form of a birth control pill right up through its current application for menopausal women in hormone replacement therapy, its use has generated enormous debate in medical journals, books, and thousands of newspaper and magazine articles.

Introduced in mid-1960, estrogen was widely touted as a "cure-all" for menopause. It was considered to be a "youth pill" that could avert twenty-six menopausal symptoms including hot flashes, osteoporosis, vaginal atrophy, sagging and shrinking breasts, wrinkles, skin cracks, chronic indigestion, absentmindedness, irritability, frigidity, depression, alcoholism, and even suicide. Not willing to let this fountain-of-youth drug pass them by, millions of women took estrogen and it became one of the top five prescription drugs in the United States.

Then in 1974, the bubble burst. Several highly respected medical studies were published linking the use of estrogen by itself to uterine cancer. Two years later, the question of estrogen's influence on breast cancer was also raised. Women dropped their prescriptions like hot potatoes, and alarms were set off at the FDA. The drug companies, which had enjoyed record profits from the sale of estrogen, very quickly got involved and what followed was a series of disputes over warning labels, patient package inserts, and legitimacy of product claims. This resulted in a more conservative approach to prescribing estrogen, with its proven benefits limited to hot flashes and vaginal dryness.

By the 1980s, a new trend emerged. Based on biochemical research, doctors began prescribing estrogen in combination with progestin to counteract the potential of uterine cancer. The FDA soon followed suit and, in 1986, revised labeling of estrogen products to include the recommendation that estrogen be taken with progestin by women who still have a uterus. Since then, research studies have linked estrogen therapy to the prevention of osteoporosis and heart disease. Prescriptions are on the rise again.

Get the Terms Straight

ERT, HRT, and OCs may not be part of your daily conversation, but these are some of the terms you need to know in order to fully understand the issues relating to hormone replacement therapy. They may seem similar, but their differences are important and worth learning. Below are some short, simple explanations.

- *Estrogen replacement therapy* (ERT) refers to the administration of low doses of estrogen given by itself to counteract some of the effects of menopause. This is often referred to as *unopposed estrogen* and is used primarily by women who no longer have a uterus.
- *Combined hormone replacement therapy* refers to the low-dose administration of two hormones, estrogen and progestin,

given in combination to counteract some of the effects of menopause.

- *Hormone replacement therapy* (HRT) is an umbrella term used to describe either estrogen or combined hormone replacement therapy and is usually used in a nonspecific or general way.
- *Progesterone* is a natural hormone that prepares the lining of the uterus for implantation of a fertilized egg.
- *Progestin* or *progestogen* is a category name and refers to substances that act like natural or synthetic progesterone. Progestin, a category of progesteronelike drugs, guards against endometrial cancer and is prescribed for women who take estrogen and still have a uterus.
- *Oral contraceptives* (OCs) are pills containing synthetic estrogen and progesterone and are used in birth control. They are usually four to five times stronger than doses used in hormone replacement therapy.

Throughout this book, the term *hormone replacement therapy* will be used to describe the topic in general, *combined hormone replacement therapy* will refer to the specific combination of estrogen and progestin, and *estrogen replacement therapy* will be used when discussing the use of estrogen by itself (unopposed estrogen).

You also may have heard about an antiestrogen drug called tamoxifen, which is administered to women with certain types of breast cancer in order to counteract the effects of menopause. This is discussed in detail in Chapter 8, "Special Problems."

Opening Pandora's Box

These are strange times. If it was the earlier part of this century, most of us in our 50s would be living our final hours on earth. In those days, menopause was less of an issue because women did not live very long after it occurred. Today, you can expect to live an average of thirty years after menopause, and medicine now provides replacements for various aging, nonfunctional, or missing parts of your body: hip replacement, kidney transplant, breast reconstruction, and, of course, hormone replacement therapy.

The issue, then, is to decide how you want to live out this extra time. One option is to consider replacing the estrogen that is no longer produced in significant amounts after menopause. In theory, this replacement will allow you to continue to benefit from some of the protective qualities estrogen provided in your younger years, which would be terrific, but at what long-term cost?

Unfortunately, there are no clear answers to the question of hormone replacement therapy and whether it is right for you. To top it off, hormone replacement therapy is a moving target, with new discoveries being made all the time. The constant barrage of new facts and figures is enough to make anyone crazy, and issues will probably not be clarified for many years to come.

Nevertheless there are several factors worth noting that may help you put the knowledge you have into perspective.

The Research Riddle

Yes, research exists on estrogen. There is even a study or two on progestin. However, the big question still remains: What impact does long-term administration of estrogen or combined hormone replacement therapy have on women's health? Right now there is no definitive answer to this question, but this is how things stand today.

KNOWN	UNKNOWN OR IN QUESTION
HEART DISEASE	
Unopposed estrogen taken orally decreases the risk of heart disease by 40–60%[a]	The effect of unopposed estrogen, delivered via patch or cream, on heart disease. The effect of progestin, given with estrogen, on reducing the risk of heart disease; some studies indicate it reverses the positive effects of estrogen.

Osteoporosis

Estrogen and combined hormone replacement therapy, taken orally or via the patch, retard osteoporotic bone loss	The effect of estrogen, delivered via vaginal cream, on osteoporotic bone loss.

Endometrial Cancer

Unopposed estrogen, taken orally, increases the risk of endometrial cancer five- to fifteenfold in women with a uterus; the addition of progestin reduces this risk to normal or better	The long-term effects of progestin.

Breast Cancer

No association has been shown with the standard dose of estrogen replacement therapy (0.625 mg) and increased risk of breast cancer[b] Long-term use of higher doses of estrogen, in any form, moderately increases the risk of developing breast cancer	The effect of estrogen at other doses or progestin on increasing breast cancer risk.

[a] Only shown by epidemiologic data using higher doses of estrogen than are currently prescribed. No clinical trials have been done.
[b] Only one study has been done that shows no increase in breast cancer risk using Premarin at this specific dosage.

Fortunately, the research community has woken up and realized there is still a great deal of work to be done in order to give women the answers they need. Despite the expense and difficulty, long-term studies are under way, but the results will not be known for many years to come. Until then, women will have to rely on the small amount of existing data to make a decision about hormone replacement therapy.

Pharmaceutical Company Influence

Drug companies are like most large American businesses—they determine a need in the market, conduct research and develop a product to fill that need, then promote it to potential buyers to make a profit on their investment. It sounds straightforward, but it is a tough, risky, and complex business, heavily regulated by the FDA. For example, it costs $200–$250 million and twelve years of research and testing to bring a new drug to market in the United States.

As you might expect, the drug companies work hard to protect their investments. Translated to your life, the drug companies that manufacture various forms of estrogen and progestin used in hormone replacement therapy have a serious vested interest in the sale of these drugs. This means that much of the information you gather is generated in one form or another by the drug companies as part of their research or promotional efforts. Typically, these companies

- Provide funding for independent research studies, the results of which are usually published in medical journals.
- Engage public relations firms to place articles related to their products in major newspapers and magazines and on television.
- Donate financial support for major medical meetings and public seminars, proceedings of which are usually covered in trade and consumer publications.
- Conduct elaborate advertising campaigns targeted at doctors and sometimes even consumers.
- Develop consumer publications on general topics, often with a bias toward their product or product category.

There is nothing wrong with any of this activity. In fact, the pharmaceutical companies are known to be some of the most sophisticated marketers in the business world. Nor is there reason to doubt the validity of information they provide. Just be aware of the source and consider the influences that may be brought to bear on the materials you read.

Hot off the Press
The media have become wizards who report news the minute it happens and deliver it to your living room in the blink of an eye.

In fact, they often scoop the medical community by reporting scientific breakthroughs announced at press conferences days and sometimes weeks before the official article, published in a medical journal, actually reaches a doctor's office.

This means that breakthroughs often hit the front page of your local newspaper and focus on the highlights of the latest discovery. Unfortunately, they are rarely reported in detail or, worse still, not put into a context with previous discoveries or ongoing research yet to be published. You are left with the headlines, confusion about what it all means, and often no professional resource to consult on the details.

Ideally, there should be a clearinghouse for medical news that would operate like the Centers for Disease Control. Run by medical professionals, this clearinghouse would release all new medical breakthroughs and position them in relation to what we already know and what is still in question. However, no such organization currently exists, nor is one currently planned. Until this happens, you need to be aware of the source of information and not panic if the news impacts your life. Be patient, wait until things settle down, and then seek out the answers you need from a well-informed professional.

> *It's scary that I can't make a choice. Every time I read an article they present one side and then the other and I can't figure out what the benefits really are. It's as if the information self-destructs.*
>
> Single woman, 48

The Hormone Replacement Therapy Research Stereotype
Although some research has been done on various aspects of hormone replacement therapy, very little of it was done using a random population sample. In most studies, research subjects are self-selected by volunteering in the first place or by choosing to join the testing cell of women slated to take hormones. What you end up with is a homogeneous group of women who share similar characteristics:

- Upper middle class.
- White.
- Advanced education (two or more years of college).
- Under regular medical care.
- A lifestyle that usually includes exercise and a good diet.
- A willingness to follow and maintain a prescribed drug regimen.

This is hardly a picture of the average American woman, and there is no question that this one-dimensional profile affects the interpretation of research results. However, if you fit this profile, you can feel confident about how the research might apply to you. Keep this in mind when reviewing studies you read about in newspapers and magazines.

Keeping Up with the Joneses

With most controversial issues, facts often get muddled by passionate beliefs on either side. You may have a friend or two already on hormone replacement therapy or perhaps have talked to other women with strong feelings on the subject. While listening to opinions can be enlightening, it is no substitute for real data. Now is the time to get some facts. Why do women decide to take hormone replacement therapy? Who are they? How long do they last on therapy? Why do they stop? How many of them are there?

Here are some tidbits to open your eyes to what women are actually thinking and doing when it comes to hormone replacement therapy.

Decision Making
In a recent study of how women make decisions about estrogen replacement therapy, researchers found most women made their decision based on their level of discomfort, primarily from hot flashes. They were much more concerned with their current problem than with any long-term risk. Some doctors report a

different picture for women who are sexually active and have concerns about vaginal atrophy. Others mentioned women's fear of specific diseases, often based on family history—cancer, heart disease, osteoporosis.

> *Unless there's a real reason to go on hormone replacement therapy, I'd just as soon avoid it. If I had symptoms I couldn't ignore, if I was tested for osteoporosis and found that I was losing bone, or there was some other compelling medical reason, I would probably do it, but I certainly wouldn't be happy about it. Mainly, I'd be afraid of breast cancer, but some of the side effects that go with hormones are also a real turnoff. I fight gaining weight all the time anyway and hormones would make it harder. I just lost a lot of weight a few years ago and I don't want to have to cope with that battle again. I also don't like putting strange substances into my body—it's that simple. It just bothers me.*
>
> Married mother, 47

In the end, it comes down to individual choice. All the statistics, odds, and reassurances in the world will never get some women over their fear of cancer. The same can be said for other women and heart disease. You will have to make the final decision by yourself. This is the only body you get and you are still in charge.

> *My gynecologist feels that hormones do help and she's studied the long-term side effects. She says women no longer sit with their shawls and knit in their middle years. She told me I was a vital woman and should do everything I could to keep that vitality and life. She strongly recommended hormones but said it was my choice in the end.*
>
> Single woman, 50

Subscribers to Therapy

Although no one knows the exact number, it is estimated that 18 percent of women over 45 years of age are on hormone replacement therapy, with a high percentage of the group coming from the upper middle class. This means 7 to 8 million women take unopposed estrogen or combined hormone replacement therapy each month. Close to 65 percent of this group (a large number of whom no longer have a uterus as a result of hysterectomy) take unopposed estrogen, with the remaining 35 percent on some form of combined therapy. A large percentage of women who fill prescriptions for hormone replacement therapy do not refill them after six months or less.

The Quitters

As appealing as hormone replacement therapy is to millions of women, the average length of therapy is between nine and twelve months. However, large numbers of women quit in less than a year for one of two reasons: They find either monthly bleeding unacceptable or the side effects from the hormones debilitating. A small number of women, usually over 60 years old, quit because they feel they no longer need the physical or psychological benefits. A few women throw in the towel in panicked response to an article in the media.

> *I hated HRT. I took estrogen and all I did was blow up like a Macy's balloon. I mean I couldn't get into my clothes and I retained water. The other terrible thing was that you went on estrogen to get rid of hot flashes and you ended up exchanging it all for having your period again. It was a vicious cycle, so I quit.*
>
> Married mother, 55

Another possible reason for discontinuing therapy is the "out of sight, out of mind" factor. The effects of heart disease and osteoporosis, two of the most compelling reasons to use hormone replacement therapy, are not easy to see. Therefore, if you are taking a drug to protect yourself from these diseases and there are no visible "improvements," it may be hard to stay the prescribed course.

There also is a hidden group of quitters, or, more correctly stated, women who never leave the starting gate. Approximately 30 percent of the women who get hormone replacement therapy prescriptions from their doctors never fill them for one reason or another. One can only assume their minds were not made up in the first place. Try to avoid this situation and take the time to make your decision clearly before you get to this point.

> *Every time I see something on hormones, I cut it out. I read it, I go back, I read it again, and I still come up with not taking them at all. I have two prescriptions for hormones in my drawer that are still lying there after three years. Both gynecologists who wrote them out said I could take them whenever I was ready. And I still haven't done anything about it.*
>
> Married woman, 51

The Facts

By now, you may be ready to give up careful decision making in favor of tossing a coin. Hang in there. Not everything associated with hormone replacement therapy is up in the air. Physicians and drug companies alike are aware of the unknowns and have done quite a bit to inject order onto chaos. For example, there are standard regimens to adhere to before prescribing; specific known benefits, risks, and side effects; and well-defined conditions that prohibit the use of hormone replacement therapy.

Unopposed Estrogen Versus Combined
Hormone Replacement Therapy

Back in the mid-1970s, physicians found an alarming increase in the incidence of uterine cancer among women who took unopposed estrogen. Research revealed that taking estrogen by itself led to a five- to fourteenfold increase in the rate of endometrial cancer due to increased buildup of the uterine lining. Since then, scientists discovered that by giving progestin, which causes the uterus to shed its lining, in combination with estrogen, the risk of developing uterine cancer became negligible.

Consequently, today the situation is straightforward. Women without a uterus are considered the primary candidates for unopposed estrogen replacement therapy. Women with a uterus are usually put on combined hormone replacement therapy with progestin.

The exception to this rule is women with a uterus who either cannot tolerate progestin or refuse to have monthly bleeding. (See The Dosing Dilemma, which appears later in this chapter, for more information on uterine bleeding.) If prodded sufficiently, doctors will prescribe unopposed estrogen to women with a uterus but often make a deal with the patient before proceeding. In this situation, doctors usually require a woman to undergo an endometrial biopsy at least once and sometimes twice every year—not a pleasant experience. Pioneered by British doctors, vaginal ultrasound, a relatively new and painless technique for monitoring the uterine lining, is now being used by some physicians throughout the country. Talk to your doctor about this alternative.

It may seem excessive, but in this situation, rigorous testing of the lining of the uterus is essential and will allow the early detection of most abnormalities and make doctor and patient alike feel confident about "breaking the rule." However, this approach is not advocated by the drug companies who manufacture estrogen or by the FDA, which approves its use.

The Benefits of Hormone Replacement Therapy

If you ask a few women on hormone replacement therapy how they feel about estrogen, you will most likely get a resoundingly positive response. In fact, many of them are evangelical in their enthusiasm and will probably try to recruit you to join their ranks. Here are some of the reasons why these women are so positive about this drug.

Hot Flashes. Hot flashes are the number one complaint of women in search of hormone replacement therapy. And it works just like magic. Hormone replacement therapy eliminates hot flashes in the majority of women, usually within two weeks. In most cases suffering and discomfort disappear and will not return unless hormone therapy is stopped. Unpredictable hot flashes will no longer wake you up in the middle of the night or catch you off guard during the day. This benefit can be achieved with all forms of hormone replacement therapy except estrogen vaginal cream, which carries too low a dose to affect hot flashes.

In addition to relief from hot flashes and night sweats, hormone replacement therapy took care of this woman's tiredness and mood swings. Her enthusiastic attitude is typical of many women, although the speed of relief may be a little questionable.

The patch has worked wonders for me. Between the fatigue, the flashes, night sweats, and mood swings, I was going nuts. Two minutes after I put on the patch, I started to feel better. No kidding . . . maybe less than two minutes, maybe fifty seconds. It was such a relief, it was unbelievable!

Married mother, 46

Vaginal Dryness. With the replacement of estrogen no longer produced by the ovaries, preliminary symptoms of vaginal atrophy like dryness, itching, and painful sexual intercourse dissipate within a few weeks. For women whose vagina is already atrophied as a result of menopause, it will take longer to restore moisture and allow the tissues to return to their previous level of pliability. However, the condition can be greatly improved with the use of hormones, and enjoyable, painless sexual activity resumed. This benefit can be achieved with estrogen vaginal cream as well as with all other forms of hormone replacement therapy.

I do think that menopause and my taking hormones have ended up having a positive effect on my sex life. I started on the estrogen patch and that didn't seem to do the trick in terms of my vaginal dryness. But when I switched to the pill, it really helped. Sex became easier, my interest improved, and I was enjoying it more. I wasn't about to give it up, no matter what. I was 35 before I actually discovered that sex could be fun. Up until then, it was like eating cardboard—I used to lie there and think of England, as they say. But then I had a climax by accident and ended up knowing a lot more about what made me feel good. Since then, it's just gotten better and better. So if all it takes is hormone therapy to keep my sexual juices flowing, then it's an easy decision for me.

Single mother, 52

Urinary Stress Incontinence. Estrogen seems to strengthen the muscles in the pelvic area including the urethra, which passes urine out of the bladder. Like the vagina, the urethra responds well to estrogen replacement by developing a thicker mucous lining and stronger surrounding muscles. Within a few weeks of taking estrogen or combined hormone replacement therapy, urinary stress incontinence usually disappears. The restoration of the tissues in this area will also guard against urinary infections. This benefit can be achieved with estrogen vaginal cream as well as with all other forms of hormone replacement therapy.

Please note: Not all urinary incontinence is brought on by menopause. It is important to see a doctor for an accurate diagnosis.

Osteoporosis. Approved by the FDA for the treatment of osteoporosis, estrogen has been found to protect against bone loss. Specifically, long-term hormone replacement therapy has been proven to prevent osteoporosis in 75 to 80 percent of women. It is especially effective in women with chemically or surgically induced menopause who have had an abrupt loss of estrogen production.

The effectiveness of hormone replacement therapy seems to center around its immediate use after the onset of menopause and its continuation for eight to ten years. Remember, this is the time period when women experience bone loss at an accelerated rate. After that, if therapy is discontinued, bone loss does resume but at a much slower rate, usually associated with the normal effects of aging. It is also important to be sure that your calcium and vitamin D intake is at the recommended level in order for hormone replacement therapy to be fully effective. This benefit can only be achieved with estrogen or combined hormone replacement therapy taken orally in dosages of 0.625 milligram or more or the transdermal estrogen patch, although recent research indicates that dosages as low as 0.45 milligram (not yet available) may work just as well. The effect of estrogen cream on osteoporotic bone loss is unknown.

This anorexic woman developed osteoporosis after years of poor diet and lack of medical care. However, she became educated about her condition, learned about the benefit of hormone replacement therapy in preventing osteoporosis, and now works hard to spread the word to other women.

> *I have osteoporosis and wasn't educated enough to do anything to prevent it. Osteoporosis means I have to limit my life in many, many ways. I can't bend; I have to be concerned about calcium. It's very burdensome and frightening. And personally, if I were to develop the advanced symptoms of it, I wouldn't want to live. That's why I feel I'm on a mission these days. I have a lot of women friends in their late 40s, and even though I try to talk to them about estrogen and osteoporosis, they don't really have a clue about the seriousness of the disease. They say, "Oh, yeah, I'm going to do something about it." But then it's a year later and they haven't.*
>
> Single woman, 53

Heart Disease. Estrogen has been shown to decrease the risk of heart disease by 40 to 60 percent. This is no mean feat, especially when you consider that heart disease is the number one cause of death in women. Although the effect is not totally understood, unopposed estrogen, delivered orally in a pill, increases the good cholesterol (HDL) by 15 to 20 percent and, at the same time, decreases the bad cholesterol (LDL) by 10 to 15 percent.

Unfortunately, this partial protection against heart disease is limited to those women who can take unopposed estrogen in pill form. Combined hormone replacement therapy does not produce the same results. In fact, progestin has been shown to reverse the positive effect on blood cholesterol.

However, new studies indicate the positive effect on cholesterol represents only 20 percent of the total heart disease benefit. The remaining 80 percent of protection is related to the blood vessels themselves. Estrogen seems to dilate blood vessels and can regress already existing plaque formation. It also seems to affect positively the architecture of the heart muscle by increasing the elasticity of the aorta.

Given this type of potentially conflicting data, it is difficult to be definitive about estrogen and heart disease. But based on existing research, most of which was done using conjugated equine estrogen (predominantly Premarin, manufactured by Wyeth-Ayerst Laboratories), the following statements hold true:

- In studies comparing women who took long-term estrogen therapy with conjugated equine estrogen against a control group, the reduction of the risk of cardiovascular disease and death from heart attack for those receiving the therapy was nearly 50 percent.
- It is unknown whether the protective effect on heart disease is as great as 50 percent when estrogen, specifically conjugated equine estrogen, is taken in combination with progesterone. Answers should be available by 1995. Current studies are also under way evaluating the effectiveness of another form of estrogen—17 β-estradiol, the primary estrogen made by the human ovary—found in Estraderm, manufactured by Ciba, and Mead Johnson's Estrace.

Mood Swings. Although it is difficult to prove as scientific fact, most women report a strong sense of well-being when taking hormone replacement therapy. Some doctors feel hormones help with PMS, which sometimes worsens as women approach menopause.

The Side Effects and Risks of Hormone Replacement Therapy

As with most positive effects, there is usually a negative side, and hormone replacement therapy is no exception. On a day-to-day basis, there are various side effects that you would expect in taking any drug. In the case of hormone replacement therapy, however, the resumption of monthly bleeding is an unappealing prospect to many women and is often classified as another side effect. Over the long term, there are also risks, some of which are clearly defined and others that are questionable but still warrant a cautionary approach. Here is the latest information on the downside.

Estrogen Side Effects. There is no real mystery about estrogen's various side effects. What is not known is how you will respond to the hormone. Everyone is different, and it is impossible to predict how comfortable you will be on the drug. Here is a list of possible side effects. None will kill you, but the presence of one or two might make you uncomfortable enough to discontinue using estrogen.

- Breast tenderness or enlargement.
- Enlargement of benign tumors of the uterus (fibroids).
- Spotty darkening of the skin, particularly on the neck and chest.

Although this woman managed to maintain her sense of humor about the side effects of hormone replacement therapy, it is clear that she was not having fun.

Estrogen therapy works pretty well for me, except every once in a while, I really seem to have side effects. Like this morning, I woke up and my breasts felt like they weighed 3,000 pounds. How am I supposed to go out there and exercise—I'll sink right through the sidewalk. This is ridiculous! Here I am 59 years old and my breasts are as sore as my pregnant daughter's.

Married mother, 59

This next woman had trouble with her weight while taking combined hormone replacement therapy, a complaint raised by many women. Although weight gain can often be traced to a change in eating or exercise habits, it can also be encouraged by taking progestin.

I've gained a few pounds and just can't lose it since I've been on estrogen. I'm not heavy, but I have gained 4 or 5 pounds that won't go away. I'll have to enroll in a new aerobics program and even though I've always exercised, I'm doing more now. If I'd eaten as well as I do now before I started taking estrogen, I'd be much slimmer. My gynecologist said that many women just can't stand the weight gain, and I have a couple of friends who are stopping because of it.

Married mother, 53

Progestational Side Effects. Progestational agents—natural progesterone or progestin—are often troublesome and side effects cause many women to drop combined hormone replacement therapy. Fortunately there are a number of different brands on the market and doctors often recommend trying several in order to find one that will not cause discomfort. Progestational side effects are similar to symptoms associated with PMS and include

- Fluid retention.
- Irritability.
- Increased appetite.
- Weight gain.
- Depression.
- Feelings of being bloated.
- Lower abdominal pressure.
- Constipation.
- Acne.

Although progestin, prescribed with estrogen, is effective in protecting women with a uterus from developing endometrial cancer, it is not approved by the FDA for this particular use. Very little is known about its effect on the body when taken for long periods of time. However, millions of women have taken progestin with no serious results other than the side effects noted above.

I can't stand the progesterone part of taking hormone replacement therapy. It's deadly for me—the first day I put that pill in my mouth I feel like I'm taking poison. It gives me terrible headaches and makes me feel all bloated and fat. It may sound crazy, but it seems like the only way to get past the side effects is to have a hysterectomy and then only take estrogen.

Married mother, 45

Endometrial Cancer. Discussed earlier in this chapter, the risk of endometrial cancer has been brought under control with the use of progestin. Women who take unopposed estrogen (without progestin) and still have a uterus have a five- to fourteenfold increased risk of developing endometrial cancer, although the cancers that do develop are usually of low stage and grade with a cure rate of about 90 percent. But who wants any form of cancer, thank you very much. Because estrogen can cause excessive cell growth in the uterus and progestin controls that growth, physicians prescribe the two together. Evidence suggests that women who take combined hormone therapy are less likely to develop endometrial cancer than women who avoid hormones completely.

The downside of this miracle for some women is the monthly bleeding brought on by progestin. Unlike your normal menstrual flow, this bleeding will usually be lighter and totally predictable and occur without cramping. Depending on your individual situation, there may be appropriate ways to avoid monthly bleeding. (See The Dosing Dilemma, which appears later in this chapter, for a more complete explanation.)

Breast Cancer. No matter how much women read about the risks of osteoporosis and heart disease, their biggest fears still center around breast cancer. Forget the statistics. If you are like most women, the thought of waking up one morning with a lump in your breast is far more real and frightening than picturing yourself with stooped posture, a broken hip, or keeling over from a heart attack. Although many women have adjusted and learned to live with breast cancer, most women are loathe to take drugs voluntarily that put them at risk, despite the known benefits.

My doctor gave me a prescription for HRT as well as some information to read provided by the drug company. Of course, it's all pro, pro, pro, but it helped me understand the history of what happened with estrogen and why it got a bad name. I really believe that with the current lower doses of estrogen and the use of progesterone you're pretty safe in terms of endometrial cancer. I think the only real question these days is breast cancer. There's no real answer, so you just have to take your best shot, do breast self-examination, and have regular mammograms.

Single mother, 45

Unfortunately, existing research on the correlation between estrogen and breast cancer is inconclusive. Consequently, there seems to be a division of opinion in the medical community with people lining up on both sides. Below is a sampling of available information:

- According to a paper published in 1991 by Trudy Bush, Ph.D., a noted epidemiologist at Johns Hopkins University, recent studies suggest the use of estrogen for more than fifteen years is associated with a moderate increase in the risk of breast cancer, but issues of research methodology and bias cloud the conclusions.
- As reported in a 1991 issue of *Archives of Internal Medicine*, combined results from multiple studies provide strong evidence that menopausal therapy consisting of 0.625 milligram or less of conjugated estrogens (Premarin) does not increase breast cancer risk.

Opinion will probably continue to waffle on this issue, but one fact remains clear: There is enough evidence out there to raise a question about the increased risk of breast cancer for women who take estrogen. There are no answers today, so you will have to make your decision based on the kind of information listed above. Another option is to roll up your sleeves, badger your doctor with questions, read everything you can get your hands on, and stay on top of the research as results of new studies are published.

> *The only danger in taking replacement therapy I've read about is breast cancer. And of course, nobody wants to take that risk. However, I've made up my mind that if I need hormones—if a doctor tells me or I'm unable to function as well—then I'll learn everything about them and give it a try. But if I don't have to, I don't think I will. On the other hand, you hear that replacement therapy protects you from heart disease. So, I end up going back and forth in my mind. I don't know if I've really formed an opinion.*
>
> Single woman, 51

Gallbladder Disease. According to the research, women who use oral estrogen after menopause are more likely to develop gallbladder disease, needing surgery, than women who do not use estrogen; the effects of estrogen via a transdermal patch are not known. Also at higher risk of developing gallstones are overweight women and mothers of several children. Consider these risk factors carefully. Gallbladder disease, while not usually fatal, can be extremely painful.

Blood Clotting. Women with a history of blood clotting should probably stay away from estrogen. For other women, previous information about increased risk of blood clotting was based on research done with high-dose oral contraceptives and women who were also smokers. New research does not support the dosages of estrogen used in hormone replacement therapy as causing an increase in blood clotting. Also, because it bypasses the liver, estrogen delivered via a patch does not appear to have any effect on blood clotting risk.

Cautionary Conditions and Contraindications
You may be knocked out of the running as a candidate even before you get a chance to make a decision on estrogen. There are several clearly defined existing conditions that warrant caution or prohibit its use.

Caution should be used with the following conditions because cyclic estrogen can make them worse:

- Seizures.
- Diabetes.
- Migraine headaches.
- History of blood clots.
- Liver disease.

The following conditions are contraindications for estrogen:

- A history of endometrial cancer.
- A history of breast cancer.
- Unexplained vaginal bleeding.
- Gallbladder disease.

I am a real candidate for breast cancer with both my mother and sister having had it. On the one hand, it was hard knowing breast cancer ran in our family. But on the other, it helped. I wouldn't touch HRT because of my family history. We don't know enough about what causes cancer, although in my case, it's clear that there's a genetic connection. I'm not in favor of hormones because they've been linked to cancer. It's just not for me.

Single woman, 43

Some words of wisdom: This is not the time to cover up any aspect of your medical history. Nor is it appropriate to try out some of your friend's hormone replacement therapy prescription. Estrogen is a natural hormone found in the body, but replacement estrogen is a drug that needs to be used safely and under the care of a physician. Take these warnings seriously.

The Dosing Dilemma

When you read a drug label, there is always a recommended dose, in theory, for everyone. Yet, no two people respond the same to drugs. In reality, the situation is often slightly different from the norm. Take a simple drug like aspirin, for example. You might take one or two aspirins for a headache but your husband may need three to get relief. He is probably bigger than you and may not respond in the same way. Your headache may be different from his. If the answer is two for you and three for him, what should the recommended dose actually be?

The questions do not stop here either. What if you have trouble swallowing pills or your pain is located close to the surface of your body? Should you try chewing Aspergum? What about aspirin in cream form? Over time, by experimenting with the standard dose, you both learn what works for your body.

Hormone replacement therapy is no different. Despite the variety of candidates for hormone replacement therapy, many physicians prescribe the standard dose to all their patients. These standard dosages are derived from research studies, but no dose has the same effect on 100 percent of the women tested. The recommendations are based on treating average symptoms and coming up with an average response. By definition, all women do not readily fall into that "average" classification.

To add to this dilemma, estrogen also comes in several forms at varying dosage levels. Moreover, there are a number of different dosing schedules available for hormone replacement therapy. This woman went through a few dosage regimens over many months before she found just the right combination to help with her hot flashes.

Hot flashes were keeping me up all night. I turned into a zombie, couldn't sleep, and was in tears most of the time. It was awful. My doctor put me on hormones, and the patch seemed to work for a while. But after about a year and a half, I started to have terribly heavy bleeding. At that point, my doctor lowered the dose and switched me to pills, and it's all working out fine. I get a period the same time every month, but it's like when I took birth control pills—very light for about three days. I never had that with the patch. It just didn't work for me.

Married mother, 53

It should come as no surprise that regulating hormone replacement therapy can be a daunting task, especially when you look at all the variables—dosage amount, drug delivery system, dosing schedule—and consider the individuality of each woman. Success is usually achieved if you and your doctor work together.

This woman was fortunate to have a doctor who understood the need for individualized dosage and gave her the support needed to stick it out until they got it right.

I asked my gynecologist about hormones and he's pretty easy to talk to. He said every woman is really unique. He doesn't care what you read in books—if you're going to take hormones, you have to give yourself a year to figure out the dosage. There are a lot of things you can do to make it more comfortable, but everybody reacts in a different way.

Married mother, 49

Pills, Patches, and Cream

These methods of drug administration, in addition to injections, are the only ones currently available in the United States for estrogen. They each have their pluses and minuses, but one of them should work for you.

Oral Estrogen. Delivered in a small pill, oral estrogen is the most widely used in hormone replacement therapy. On the plus side, for most women it is easy and convenient to take.

On the minus side, the pill has to pass through the digestive tract and be processed by the liver in order to enter the bloodstream. Some of the estrogen may be lost during digestion or it may not be absorbed into the bloodstream at a constant rate. This causes peaks and valleys of estrogen in the bloodstream, which may result in side effects. Because some of the estrogen is lost during the digestive process, higher doses must be taken in order to be effective.

The Transdermal Patch. Since its introduction several years ago, the skin patch has been welcomed as an alternative to oral estrogen. Almost two inches in diameter, or slightly larger depending on dosage, the patch looks like a cellophane disk with an adhesive backing. You put it on just like a Band-Aid anywhere on your body that is comfortable, except for your breast. It needs to be changed twice a week, and you must vary the location each time, allowing at least a week before using the same site again. Bathing, swimming, or showering will not affect the patch.

On the plus side, it is a boon to women who have difficulty swallowing pills or remembering to take medication on a daily basis. Because the estrogen enters the bloodstream through the skin, it does not have to pass through the digestive tract and the liver. This results in an even and continuous flow of estrogen directly into your bloodstream, reducing or eliminating potential side effects. Smaller doses of estrogen can be used because of this direct delivery route. It is also suitable for women with clotting problems, as this delivery system seems to eliminate the problem.

On the negative side, the patch can cause redness and skin irritation at the application site for some women. In humid climates, it can also be difficult to keep in place. It is unclear whether the patch offers the same protection against heart disease as the pill.

Estrogen Vaginal Cream. Used primarily to reverse vaginal dryness and urinary stress incontinence, estrogen cream is applied directly to the vagina using a small applicator that comes with the product. The typical dose is 1 gram applied twice a week. It is extremely effective in dealing with vaginal dryness and urinary incontinence and delivers a relatively low dose of estrogen. Vaginal cream is especially attractive to women who are interested in treating only dryness and incontinence. It is also suitable for women with clotting problems, as this delivery system seems to eliminate the problem.

On the minus side, it is unappealing to women who are uncomfortable touching themselves or using tampons. Care needs to be taken in application to make sure you only use the proper dosage. Because of the relatively small dose of estrogen, vaginal cream will usually not relieve hot flashes or provide other benefits associated with the prevention of osteoporosis and heart disease. In some patients, where other dosage forms are not acceptable or cause side effects, doctors may prescribe larger amounts of vaginal cream to provide enough estrogen to relieve hot flashes and other menopausal signs.

Some words of warning: Although the majority of the dose of vaginal estrogen is delivered locally, some amount is also absorbed systemically and circulates throughout the body; women with absolute estrogen contraindications should not use it at all. Also, when you use estrogen vaginal cream, you are taking unopposed estrogen. This means women who still have a uterus must be alert to the risk of endometrial cancer. If you bleed when using estrogen cream, you must see your doctor right away. It probably means you are taking enough estrogen through the cream to actually build up a lining in your uterus. Once that lining is built up, it must be shed in order for your uterus to remain healthy. Your doctor will probably prescribe progestin to make sure this happens. More than likely, you will only have to take progestin on an intermittent basis to make sure you shed any built-up uterine lining. Remember, although estrogen cream is only applied to the vagina, it does have an effect on your entire system. You must be careful and give it the respect you would any drug you take into your body.

Estrogen Injections. Certainly not first on most women's list, estrogen is available by injection. For relief from hot flashes and other symptoms, you can get injections once a month and never have to think about it anymore. On the negative side, injections require a visit to the doctor each month. Delivery of the drug is not gradual and often causes side effects.

The Bleeding Question

One of the most difficult things to understand about hormone replacement therapy is when you will bleed, how much, and for how long. The answers are more predictable than you might expect. Of course, bleeding patterns will vary based on the individual, but there are some basic concepts that apply in most cases:

- If you do not have a uterus, you will not bleed. Whether or not you still have your ovaries is irrelevant in terms of bleeding.
- If you have a uterus and take combined cyclical therapy—estrogen for twenty-five consecutive days and progesterone for ten to twelve consecutive days—you will have light bleeding every month for two to five days. It will usually be completely predictable and occur within twenty-four to forty-eight hours after taking your last progestin pill. After a few years, even this light monthly bleeding will stop, as the lining of your uterus becomes nonfunctional. However, you will still need to continue to take progesterone, even without your monthly periods.
- If you have a uterus and are on continuous combined therapy—estrogen and progestin taken every day—you will go through a four- to six-month time span of unpredictable breakthrough bleeding, after which all bleeding will stop. The majority of women on continuous therapy have no bleeding after nine months.

This describes "normal" bleeding on hormone replacement therapy. Any other bleeding is not and should be taken quite seriously. Do not ignore it and hope it will disappear next month. This is a clear signal that things may not be right, and you must see a doctor right away.

Bleeding on estrogen therapy has not bothered me a bit. A lot of women say they don't want to have their periods again, but it's really not a big deal when you're on estrogen. If anything, it's made me feel younger because I'm still buying Tampax.

Married mother, 53

How to Take Your Medicine

Whether you opt for the pill or the patch, take estrogen unopposed or with progestin, you have a choice of two basic schedules—cyclical or continuous. Cyclical therapy, designed to imitate the normal menstrual cycle, is the schedule physicians have used for many years. Both estrogen and progestin typically were stopped for five days every month. Newer approaches typically use estrogen every day and cycle only the progestin for ten to twelve days a month.

Continuous therapy using both estrogen and progestin, relatively new and considered experimental by some doctors, was created to give a constant supply of hormones and completely avoid monthly uterine bleeding.

Here is how these regimens work.

	SCHEDULE AND STANDARD DOSE	UTERINE BLEEDING
CYCLICAL		
Estrogen therapy (unopposed)	Estrogen for 25 consecutive days Pill: 0.625 mg conjugated equine estrogen or 1 mg 17 β-estradiol Patch: 0.05 or 0.1 mg	None for women without a uterus; several days for women with a uterus (not recommended), beginning on day 26
Combined therapy	Estrogen for 25 consecutive days; progestin for 10–12 consecutive days beginning on day 16; 5 days without hormones beginning on day 26 Pill: 0.625 mg conjugated equine estrogen or 1 mg 17 β-estradiol *plus* 5 mg progestin Patch: 0.05 or 0.1 mg estrogen *plus* 5 mg oral progesterone	Several days beginning on day 26; bleeding usually stops after a few years

THE INSIDE STORY: Cyclical therapy is well suited for women who have just started menopause and are not uncomfortable with monthly bleeding. Unlike your premenopausal menstrual periods, monthly bleeding on combined hormone replacement therapy is much lighter and usually lasts only a few days. Most women do not have cramping. Your monthly bleeding will be completely predictable and you will have a strong feeling of control.

Many physicians start women on cyclical therapy at the beginning of the month, probably to make it easier to remember. If you play that scenario out, you can plan on having a period every Thanksgiving, Christmas, and probably New Year's Eve. Or you can start your thirty-day cycle in a way to better fit your lifestyle. It does not matter when you start the cycle, but you must take your hormones at the right time and for the prescribed number of days.

Determined to make hormone replacement therapy work just when she wanted it to, this woman insisted on changing the initial routine her doctor had prescribed for her.

At the beginning, I was put on the estrogen pill for most of the month, days 1 to 25, and on the fifteenth of the month I took progesterone for ten days. That meant that my period came like clockwork on the twenty-fifth of each month and I would then wait until the first of the month to begin the regimen all over again. Well, I'm a bookkeeper, and the twenty-fifth of each month is when I have the heaviest workload. The last thing I need is my period at that time. So my doctor has changed my routine so that I get my period around the ninth or tenth and it's made all the difference."

Married mother, 56

	SCHEDULE AND STANDARD DOSE	UTERINE BLEEDING
CONTINUOUS		
Estrogen therapy (unopposed)	Estrogen every day Pill: 0.625 mg conjugated equine estrogen or 1 mg 17 β-estradiol	None for women with a uterus

	SCHEDULE AND STANDARD DOSE	UTERINE BLEEDING
Combined therapy	Estrogen every day, progestin every day Pill: 0.625 mg conjugated equine estrogen or 1 mg 17 β-estradiol *plus* 2.5 mg progestin Patch: 0.05 or 0.1 mg estrogen *plus* 2.5 mg oral progestin	Unpredictable breakthrough bleeding for 4–6 months (sometimes longer); bleeding stops after adjustment period

THE INSIDE STORY: Continuous therapy is considered experimental for two reasons. First, although estrogen and progesterone occur throughout the month in a normal menstrual cycle, their levels fluctuate significantly during an average twenty-eight-day cycle. With continuous therapy, hormonal levels remain constant. Second, no one knows the effects of long-term estrogen and progestin use. However, many women take continuous therapy with no ill effects.

Many women turn to continuous combined therapy to avoid monthly bleeding. For most women, continuous doses of estrogen and progestin will work eventually to stop all uterine bleeding. However, many women cannot hang in long enough to get past the four- to six-month transition period of unpredictable breakthrough bleeding that goes with the territory. It can be uncomfortable, inconvenient, and troubling. Depending on the amount of bleeding, your doctor may monitor your uterine lining with a biopsy or vaginal ultrasound to make sure everything is all right.

Sometimes it helps to understand what is going on during continuous combined therapy. You might want to flip back to Chapter 2 to refresh your memory about the workings of hormones during the menstrual cycle. Basically, estrogen stimulates the growth of the lining of the uterus and progesterone helps additional blood vessels form in that lining to make it ready for pregnancy. When the progesterone is removed, the lining sheds in the form of menstrual bleeding. With continuous therapy, you take both estrogen and progestin all the time. After several months, your body starts to adjust to both hormones, less uterine lining is produced, and the uterus eventually shrinks and atrophies. The result: no more uterine bleeding.

Continuous therapy is best suited for older women, in their late 50s and early 60s, whose uterus has probably already atrophied and who most likely will not experience much breakthrough bleeding, if any, during the transition time. Other candidates are women with the patience and commitment to make it through the transition period and a compelling desire to be on hormone replacement therapy without the side effect of withdrawal bleeding.

Going the Distance

Finding the right type of hormone replacement therapy gives new meaning to the word *personalization*. The same can be said for determining how long you should stay on hormones once you begin. There is no hard and fast rule. Some women stay on therapy just a few years to alleviate hot flashes. Others, who are at high risk for osteoporosis, may opt for longer-term therapy.

It all depends on what you want to get out of hormone replacement therapy. Sometimes it may be appropriate to change your therapy after a certain time period. For example, you may start out with oral therapy for hot flashes and later, when you seem to be past them, switch over to vaginal cream to gain continual relief from vaginal dryness.

When talking to friends about their dosage regimens, it is helpful to remember just how individual hormone replacement therapy can be. This woman's circle of friends is a perfect example of the range of treatment.

I have a few really close friends and we often talk about menopause and hormones. There are four of us who are on four completely different kinds of dosages, although one friend raises and lowers her dosage depending on what everyone else is doing. One takes them for twenty-eight days straight; I take them for three weeks, then one week off; another one has the patch; and the last one is not taking any progesterone. And we take hormones for different reasons, too. One of us has serious heart disease in her family—both of her parents died from it; another one had terrible hot flashes; and my closest friend had a hysterectomy ten years ago.

Single mother, 53

Whether you take hormones for only a few months or stay on therapy for many years, the key to success is understanding all of the variables, complying with instructions, and having patience, patience, patience. If you are truly committed to the potential benefits, you will be able to find a way to make hormone replacement therapy work. Explore all the options and keep trying until you get it right.

If You Decide Yes

Like most desirable things in life, therapy often has strings attached. If you decide to take hormone replacement therapy, you are obligated to follow a routine of regular medical checkups. Although you alone are responsible for your decision, it is important to enter into a partnership with your physician to ensure your continued good health. All doctors who prescribe hormone replacement therapy have a set of standard procedures to be followed with each patient, depending on their health and choice of therapy. These follow-up examinations are mandatory, and unless you are prepared to comply with your doctor's requirements, you should not opt for hormone replacement therapy.

Most doctors see their hormone replacement therapy patients at least twice a year. You may have to go more often during the first year in order to properly adjust your dosage. Your initial visit will include most or all of the following: pelvic examination; Pap smear; breast exam; mammogram; family history; bone density test to determine baseline; and blood tests to measure cholesterol, blood sugar, hormone, and calcium levels.

Examination procedures during follow-up visits vary according to your health but often include pelvic examination, Pap smear, breast exam, mammogram (annually), vaginal ultrasound, endometrial biopsy (if appropriate), and more blood tests. Interim visits may be necessary in order to regulate hormone dosage and control any existing side effects.

Seeing a physician this often may be a new experience for you. View it as an opportunity to take an active role in your health care. The partnership you establish with your doctor during hormone replacement therapy is an excellent model for the kind of relationship that should exist for all your medical care. It only works if you maintain an open dialogue and are honest in your communications.

What Happens When You Stop

Possible Scenarios

As they say, "The wheel goes round and round and where it stops, nobody knows." What will happen when you stop taking hormones is not quite this chancy, but the answers are far from crystal clear. Again, each woman responds differently.

Remember, women take hormone replacement therapy for an average of nine to twelve months. This is a short amount of time and hormones do not have a long-lasting effect on the body. Although there are no hard and fast rules about what to expect when you stop therapy, here are some possible scenarios:

- *If severe hot flashes and vaginal dryness prompted you to take hormones*, and you took them for less than a year, there is a good chance they will return when you stop therapy. Many physicians suggest a gradual tapering-off process, which makes a difference for many women. However, the end result is usually the same.
- *If you started hormone replacement therapy with mild hot flashes or vaginal dryness*, these symptoms might return when you quit, but they disappear for about 80 percent of women after a few months.

- *If you took combined hormone replacement therapy and quit,* your monthly bleeding will also disappear. You may have a one- or two-month adjustment period, but assuming you were menopausal when you started therapy, you should not have any bleeding after you stop.
- *If you started hormone replacement therapy within a year or two of the onset of menopause, and you quit after a few years or less,* you can expect to experience rapid bone loss in much the same way you would have without therapy. Protection from the risk of osteoporosis will stop when you stop therapy.
- *If you started hormone replacement therapy within a year or two of the onset of natural menopause and stayed on it for more than six years before quitting,* you probably will have gained protection from the initial rapid bone loss associated with the onset of menopause. However, protection from bone loss associated with the natural aging process will disappear when you stop taking hormones. (See Chapter 3, "Postmenopause," for more information on osteoporosis.)
- *If you quit therapy at any time,* protection against the risk of heart disease will also be eliminated.

When to Throw In the Towel

You might be part of the minority of women who take hormone replacement therapy for many years and wonder when they should quit. Again, there is no hard and fast rule, and with the lack of research on long-term estrogen use, you really are on your own. One serendipitous approach is to use the average age of death in women as a benchmark. Working backward from age 78, allow twelve to fourteen years for the development of clinically significant osteoporosis, and you come up with a quitting age of 65. However, what happens if you are going to live to be 105?

There are no easy answers, and there is nothing terrible about quitting therapy. Just make sure you know why you are quitting so that you avoid starting and stopping all over again.

The Big Decision

Whether or not to take hormone replacement therapy is a personal decision. It is also an extremely difficult one to make with the available information, but it is a decision you must make, one way or the other.

If you have read all of this chapter, you have an understanding of estrogen and what it can and cannot do. You know the benefits and the side effects of hormone replacement therapy and are aware of the different options for taking it. You also have a grasp of the existing research, what we know today, and what is still in question.

Now it is time to use this knowledge, put all the pieces of the puzzle on the table, and figure out how to put them together. Many physicians and other people often refer to this as a *risk–benefit analysis*. The term seems inappropriate and slightly cavalier given the serious implications of your decision—one that you are forced to make based on limited information. This process may feel very much like a numbers game, but remember you are an individual, not a statistic. You need to be confident that you are doing the best you can for your body, so take the time to think this decision through very carefully.

Having made her decision not to take hormone replacement therapy, this woman still had her doubts. With the lack of definitive information, she understandably continued to long for some ongoing support from the medical community.

My decision not to take HRT frightens me in a way: Am I making a mistake? Or are the women who are taking it making a mistake? We don't know enough about it right now, and it's going to take my generation and maybe another one to find out if there are any problems. I rationalize my decision by thinking HRT is not nature's way. In fact, it just might be a big scheme by the pharmaceutical companies, especially when you look at the monthly cost of taking this drug for the rest of your life. I had an interesting conversation with a young doctor just out of medical school who had a refreshing approach to taking HRT. She feels that women need to educate themselves more and gives her patients a reading list, pro and con, and supports them in their decision—no matter what they choose to do. Hopefully that kind of attitude is the wave of the future.

Married mother, 50

Opinions from the Experts

While you rack your brain over this decision, the experts on drugs and women's health are caught in a similar bind. They must grapple with the same limited information, formulate opinions, and then state publicly how they stand on hormone replacement therapy. Unlike you, however, they have access to some of the best minds in the world and hear testimony from experts on a regular basis. Although you may not subscribe to opinions of the FDA or the American College of Obstetricians and Gynecologists, it is interesting to know their thinking on the subject.

In June 1991, the FDA met to examine the risk–benefit ratio of combined estrogen and progestin therapy and determine whether it was low enough to warrant the review of specific new drug applications for a combined drug. Expert testimony was presented, and the advisory committee developed the following opinions:

- Virtually all premenopausal women could be candidates for either estrogen replacement or combined hormone replacement therapy.
- Unopposed estrogen raises the uterine cancer risk after one year; breast cancer becomes a question after ten years; cardiovascular protection appears to be indefinite.
- Progestins, administered more than ten days each month, reduce the uterine cancer risk.
- There is sufficient data on the risk–benefit assessment of hormone replacement therapy for women with an intact uterus to justify long-term treatment.
- There are insufficient data to determine the impact of progestins on breast cancer.

- There are insufficient data to determine the impact of progestins on coronary heart disease.
- There is insufficient information for specific estrogen and progestin compounds, doses, and regimens affecting the risk–benefit assessment.
- The issues are sufficiently resolved for the FDA to consider approval of specific new drug applications for combined hormone replacement therapy.

Looking at the subject from a different angle, the American College of Obstetricians and Gynecologists offers the following advice to physicians in their treatment of patients:

At present, there are insufficient data to indicate that all postmenopausal women must be treated with estrogen replacement. For that reason, the benefits and risks, as they pertain to each patient, should be reviewed with her in detail. Ultimately, it is the patient who must decide and give her informed consent.

As a final note, the National Women's Health Network views the issue from an entirely different perspective. Supported by individual and organizational members representing over 500,000 women, the network accepts no financial support from pharmaceutical companies. In a position paper on taking hormones and women's health, prepared by the staff and board of the network with the assistance of menopause activists, researchers, nurses, and physicians, they state their views unequivocably.

We object to the view of normal menopause as a deficiency disease. Menopause does not automatically require "treatment."

We are critical of the routine prescribing of hormones for healthy women because of the known risks associated with the drugs used and the lack of complete data on risks and benefits. These drugs are potent and may increase the possibility of users developing some cancers and other diseases.

Some Perspectives on Risk

Before you start rearranging the puzzle pieces, you need to understand the concept of risk. If you are not a statistician or a professional researcher, it is easy to get confused about what all the percentages signify. It can be even more difficult to put all these figures into some sort of meaningful perspective. Take the following example: A 200 percent increase in the risk of a rare disease may not be nearly as important to you as a 10 percent decrease in the risk of a common one. Or, if you are at low risk for a specific disease, an increase of 30 percent risk may not be significant to you. It is important to understand the risk and then be able to apply it to your own situation.

Dr. Lee Goldman and Dr. Anna Tosteson of Brigham and Women's Hospital in Boston calculated some absolute risks, the actual risk of suffering or dying from an illness, and came up with the following.

Women over 50 have a

31 percent risk of dying from heart disease.
2.8 percent risk of dying from breast cancer.
2.8 percent risk of a hip fracture.
0.7 percent risk of endometrial cancer.

Looking at these same issues from another perspective, Dr. Trudy Bush, an epidemiologist at Johns Hopkins, expressed risk this way.

For every 2,000 postmenopausal women:

20 will develop heart disease.
6 will develop breast cancer.
11 will develop severe bone loss.
3 will develop endometrial cancer.

This is not a strict comparison of apples to apples, but presented from two different angles, it can help you get your arms around the issues.

Your Needs, Expectations, and Requirements
Take a hard look at your concerns about menopause and the
physical changes you are going through. Think about the health
history of your family and be honest about your attitude toward
osteoporosis, heart disease, and breast cancer. Examine how you
take care of your body on a regular basis in terms of preventive
medical care, eating, and exercise. Ask yourself a lot of questions:

- Are hot flashes making you crazy? Are they conflicting with
  your day-to-day ability to function?
- What's happening with your sex life? Is intercourse painful?
- What are your greatest fears about aging? What impact
  does menopause have on them?

Now come up with ten more questions of your own. Consider
the answers carefully and you will begin to understand the level
of your need for hormone replacement therapy.

Next, assuming you have a need for therapy, make a list of
what you expect it to do for you. Pick up a pen and take five
minutes to write it all down. Look at your list and cross out
anything that does not appear to be realistic, like no wrinkles, no
cholesterol worries, or no sagging breasts. What remains should
be a reasonable picture of what hormone replacement therapy
means to you personally. With this personalized perspective, you
are in a good position to meet with a physician to discuss the
prospect of therapy. If you are still unsure, continue to ask the
hard questions of yourself and others who may be helpful.

Finally, review the requirements for taking hormone replacement therapy:

- Medication daily or twice a week.
- Addition of progesterone if you still have your uterus.
- Possible monthly bleeding.
- Initial medical exam.
- Follow-up medical exams every six months.

Can you remember to take medication? Will you be rigorous about seeing your doctor? Are you willing to go the distance to make sure you are comfortable with your dosage? What about having your period again? This is the reality of taking hormone replacement therapy. Make sure you understand it.

The only way to be successful with therapy is to set clear goals, be honest about what to expect, and get comfortable with the required medical regimen. This is tough and will require a lot of work on your part. In the end, this exercise will be worth the effort and you will be certain of making the best possible decision.

Chapter Five

Alternative Treatment

As a student in the 1960s, I came to think of anything labeled "alternative" as far out, rebellious, and off the wall. Since then, society has loosened up a bit. Although the term "alternative" is still charged with some of that antiestablishment electricity, it is now part of the mainstream vocabulary used to indicate another choice or, more commonly, a nonorthodox option.

Although there is a wide range of available alternatives, the focus in this chapter is on those considered to be mainstream, specifically relevant to menopause, and easily accessible. This is not the place to learn about soaking herbs for twenty-four hours in order to produce a hormone derivative or special meditation practices to alleviate stress. Instead you will discover readily available therapies proven to work for large numbers of women over time.

People turn to alternative treatment for a variety of reasons—frustration with conventional medical practices, lack of results, desire for more control, attraction to natural medications. This woman's attitude is typical of many who swear by a nontraditional approach to health care.

I have been seeing alternative doctors for years and wouldn't have it any other way. They are very caring and nonjudgmental. They also do not make decisions for me or give me ultimatums telling me this is the only solution for my problem. With these doctors, I have real choices. I truly participate in my own health care.

Married mother, 52

As positive as this sounds, if you opt for alternative treatment, you will have to contend with a rigorous search to find hard, cold scientific data for many prescribed natural remedies. Unlike traditional prescription drugs, most substances used in alternative treatment are not patented and are in the public domain. This means that the potential for financial gain, which usually drives drug companies to sponsor significant medical research, just does not exist. Although good scientific data can be found, it is usually published in scientific studies that rarely appear in mainstream medical journals or consumer publications. With that in mind, I have gathered information from fully accredited and highly respected physicians who also offer more traditional forms of treatment to their patients. Much of the information is anecdotal but represents years of positive results with women going through menopause.

Alternative Treatment Approaches

Alternative approaches to standard medical care are all over the map, but complementary medicine, homeopathy, Chinese herbal medicine, and acupuncture are four of the most highly regarded and popular options available. Each one is different but they all share a common philosophy: Treat the patient, not the disease.

According to Dr. Leo Galland, who practices complementary medicine in New York City, "Conventional medicine basically asks what disease does the patient have and then treats the disease. A good physician will make allowances for the individuality of the patient, but fundamentally it's a matter of diagnosing the disease and treating the disease." Practitioners of alternative medicine take a different tact and try to figure out what is going on with the patient as a whole organism. Galland explains, "The treatment that's implemented is aimed at correcting whatever disturbances are found in the individual, with the notion that if you correct these imbalances and disturbances, the patient can then overcome the disease on her own."

With this scenario, alternative practitioners still use the patient's complaints but also gather additional data to make their diagnosis by looking at skin, nails, and hair—key indicators of the state of nutrition and metabolism—and assessing lifestyle and pertinent emotional issues. It is this comprehensive approach that truly distinguishes alternative medicine.

According to Dr. Serafina Corsello, who practices complementary medicine in New York City, "The traditional medical world does not have a comprehensive approach to treatment. We have made a disastrous change of course and have gone from treating the whole person to the treatment of the right or left pinky finger. The practitioners who have revolted and moved from the particular back to the whole person are the alternative or complementary physicians. These doctors represent the return to the balance. In this balance, a person is the sum of the whole, which often represents more than the mathematical sum of the various parts. For example, while spiritual malaise can do much harm to the whole body, a well-balanced individual can handle a diseased organ and even regenerate it."

Complementary Medicine

Complementary medicine, also known as holistic medicine, is a prime example of this patient-centered approach in both diagnosis and treatment. Based on the premise that all the healing arts can be made to complement one another, it can include nutritional medicine, herbal therapies, acupuncture, stress management, and homeopathy. Practiced only by licensed physicians, complementary medicine first and foremost stresses nontoxic, noninvasive interventions. As a secondary alternative and only if necessary, complementary physicians may also employ conventional methods of treatment such as blood tests, X rays, prescription medication, and surgery.

Over the years, many of these nonconventional treatments have been so successful that they are now part of the standard traditional medical repertoire. For example, use of what were formerly considered megadoses of vitamins, particularly vitamins C and E, is now widespread. Furthermore, mainstream physicians now tout the benefits of magnesium and fatty acids, which as recently as twelve years ago were ignored by the traditional medical community. Even Harvard Medical School is propounding some of the strategies of complementary medicine and recently offered an extensive seminar on the use of nutrition for the treatment and prevention of disease. Consequently, many experts believe complementary medicine is the leading edge of tomorrow's conventional medical practice.

Homeopathy
Developed in the early 1800s by German physician and chemist Samuel Hahnemann, homeopathy is often referred to as the grandfather of alternative medical techniques. It is a unique system of medical treatment based on the principle of administering tiny doses of natural substances in order to stimulate a patient's internal healing mechanisms. Homeopathic medications are derivatives of natural plants, minerals, and animal substances diluted to an extreme degree in order to avoid toxicity and side effects. According to Dr. Michael B. Schachter in his article "Classical Homeopathy," which appeared in the summer/fall 1990 issue of *Health Letter of the Foundation for the Advancement of Innovative Medicine*, "The major advantages of homeopathy include the avoidance of side effects from conventional drugs, the ability of homeopathic medications to successfully treat a variety of health problems simultaneously, and its potential to strengthen the patient's internal defenses, thus helping to prevent future illness."

One of the key elements of homeopathy is an extensive patient interview. Unlike a conventional medical history, which usually covers symptoms and problems, the homeopathic interview emphasizes internal or external factors that may have an influence on your complaint. Questions about your emotional and mental states are important as well as any preferences you have for specific foods or room temperature. A good homeopath will also be concerned about all aspects of your day-to-day existence that impact your lifestyle and your health.

> *My first visit was two hours long, and my homeopath investigated my history in terms of health, emotional problems, what I ate, how I slept, how I felt about things, whether I liked my husband—just my entire self, everything about my being. We are not just a liver or a lung or a breast, and it's important that we look at our entire being as far as our health is concerned.*
>
> Married mother, 55

An individualized approach to health care is appealing to many people and this well-traveled woman found homeopathy to be a logical choice for her ongoing medical needs.

> *I first became interested in homeopathy when I was living in London and had a very bad back. The English are very supportive of homeopathy; it's something that everyone uses to one degree or another. After successful treatment of my back, I became less enamored of conventional medicine, how it's used, and the fact that everyone is given the same medication. It just seems to me that everybody is different and should be treated as an individual. It's the customized treatment that makes me really like homeopathy.*
>
> Single mother, 52

Classical homeopaths use only one homeopathic medication at a time, delivered in the form of small sugar pellets or liquid drops taken orally. There are two basic approaches to dosage recommendations: Either a single high-potency dose of the selected remedy is given, followed by a four- to five-week waiting period before reevaluation, or low dosages of the appropriate remedy are administered on a daily basis.

Many patients undergoing homeopathic treatment develop a temporary increase in symptoms before they begin to improve. Generally lasting from a few hours to a few days, the temporary increase in symptoms is usually an indication that the correct remedy was selected. As you might expect, increased symptoms tend to be more severe with higher dosages. If an improper remedy is prescribed, the patient will usually have no reaction at all.

The real art of homeopathy is combining the knowledge of the patient's symptoms with significant lifestyle factors to determine the appropriate remedy. However, patient participation in this process is also key. Dr. Judyth Reichenberg-Ullman, a naturopathic physician in Seattle specializing in homeopathy, emphasizes the need for patient commitment in order to get the most out of your treatment. "Homeopathy isn't a method of healing that requires only a single visit. It's really a process, and to make the most of it, you need to give it at least six months and preferably a year or two. After all, the purpose of homeopathy is profound healing of the whole person on mental, physical, and emotional levels. The results that someone will get with homeopathy from just one visit, as compared to really sticking with it over time, are remarkably different. You can expect deep psychological change, as well as changes in your physical symptoms—even ones you've had for years."

Although most homeopaths emphasize long-term commitment, they also note that many results, especially for menopausal complaints, can be achieved within a month or so. As a general rule, homeopathy is usually effective for most people. This woman was pleasantly surprised when she sought out a homeopath for the first time in order to cope with some of her menopausal problems.

I had hot flashes to a small degree, but my biggest problem was the emotional roller coaster ride I was experiencing day in and day out. I was an absolute monster. I'd yell at the people I worked with and fight with my best friend for no reason at all. I just wasn't myself. Hormones aren't for me—I don't think they're natural—but I felt I needed something to get myself back on track and be a person everyone could live with. My daughter, who is a premed student, gave me several articles to read about homeopathy, so I thought I'd give it a try. At first, it sounded like witchcraft, but after some investigation, it started to make sense—the concept of getting your whole life force in order and back on track was very appealing. The biggest stepping-stone was when my homeopathic doctor asked me to give up coffee—I'd already given up cigarettes, so this wasn't much fun. But I feel more in control this way and it's much better than going to conventional doctors who wanted me to take all those pills. The remedy prescribed was subtle, but it worked. I'm no longer fighting with my friends, the people at work say that I'm really much nicer, and my patience is back. All in all, my temperament is more like it used to be. I have more energy and feel more positive about life in general.

Single woman, 56

Dr. Reichenberg-Ullman has found homeopathy to be effective at least 80 percent of the time in treating menopausal women, but the remedies prescribed for each are as different as the women themselves. Not all women complaining of hot flashes receive the same treatment. Because the practice of homeopathy is so individualized, it is not uncommon for Dr. Reichenberg-Ullman to use up to fifteen different homeopathic remedies to treat a group of thirty to forty menopausal women.

The following examples of several homeopathic remedies along with the personal profile of the patient's situation will give you a clearer picture of the individualized nature of their application and effect. Menopausal women with very specific complaints found relief shortly after taking the prescribed homeopathic remedy. However, although immediate relief might occur, it is unclear whether homeopathic remedies provide long-term protection from conditions like osteoporosis. If you choose to use homeopathy, it is important to continue regular monitoring of your bone density and lipid profiles.

Patient profile	Menstrual periods few and far between, awakened regularly at 3:00 A.M. feeling hot and uncomfortable, skin rashes, tendency to feel hot easily, fear of heights, lots of energy, good sex, 49 years old.
Homeopathic remedy	Sulfur
Patient profile	Hot flashes, touchy, impatient, no desire for sex, no motivation, constipation, constantly grazed on pickles, 50 years old.
Homeopathic remedy	Sepia
Patient profile	Hot flashes, personality change, edgy, restless sleep, flew off the handle for no reason, onset of menstrual periods lessened the intensity of these complaints, 52 years old.
Homeopathic remedy	Lachesis

Homeopathy is an art. It requires knowledge, experience, and good listening skills on the part of the practitioner. It also demands commitment, responsibility, and trust on the part of the patient. There is no room for self-treatment in homeopathy, especially when dealing with menopause. Homeopathy is one alternative form of treatment that is a true partnership between you and your doctor.

Chinese Herbal Medicine and Acupuncture
The oldest recorded form of medicine still in existence, Chinese herbal medicine dates back to 3000 to 2500 B.C. when two great emperors, ruling within 500 years of each other, wrote detailed treatises on their philosophies and discoveries about the body and how it works. Legend has it that Shen Nung, the older of the

two emperors, was born with a glass stomach, which enabled him to watch everything that was happening inside and determine its positive or negative effect. Whether or not you believe in his see-through stomach, Shen Nung was probably the first nutritionist and wrote about more than 200 herbs and plants, carefully documenting their properties and effects. These writings have been handed down through the years, tested, retested, and augmented to form the basis of Chinese medicine as it is practiced today.

Reliance on herbs and other natural substances can be a satisfying alternative to more traditional Western medicine. With her interest in Chinese medicine, this woman developed a different attitude about the effects of herbs on her changing body as she experienced menopause.

> *The one thing that makes me very comfortable with the herbs that I'm taking is that they restimulate your own hormonal response. Therefore, you're not really replacing hormones, as you would with standard hormone replacement therapy. Instead, your body is being encouraged to do what is normal for you. And frankly, within a couple of months of treatment, I felt just like my old self.*
> Married mother, 47

Radically different from its Western counterpart, Chinese medicine is based on the concept that the body must be in harmony with the world as it goes through different stages of life. The Chinese believe the body has a meridian system—a series of riverlike channels through which *chi*, loosely translated as "energy," flows. There are twelve interconnected rivers that share a circadian rhythm of the flow of *chi*. It is difficult to reduce this complex philosophy to a quick overview, but simply put, if the *chi* flows properly, then a person remains healthy.

Dr. Serafina Corsello eloquently describes the positive effect of working within this Eastern philosophy. "You have to balance the energy forces to promote healing—first comes the energy and then comes the forces of biochemistry. I see the body as an electrical grid, which I call the 'template of healing.' It's like a metallic mesh with lines, called *meridians*, going up and down. Where the lines intersect with the horizontals, those are the points of resistance to the transport of energy flowing up and down to the various organs. If you facilitate the transport of energy, its flow stimulates proper biochemical reactions and restores organ integrity. This is the true healing effect."

One of the twelve channels of energy is called "the three heaters" and controls the harmonization and integration of respiration, digestion, and elimination—the basic metabolic system. Irregularities in the flow of *chi* indicate metabolic imbalances that require adjustment. In order to control menstrual regularity and help women with symptoms associated with menopause, Chinese doctors often focus their efforts on the three heaters, prescribing various herbal compounds or acupuncture treatments known to regulate this channel.

Acupuncture is the practice of inserting extremely thin needles into various areas of the body. Using the theory of *chi*, an acupuncturist will insert a series of needles at the junctions of the appropriate meridians. Devotees of acupuncture say the needles are virtually painless and, in fact, are calming and relaxing.

> *I find acupuncture very restful and reassuring. There's absolutely no pain involved and you spend your twenty- or thirty-minute session just lying there. It's obviously a quiet time while the needles do their work. You don't feel the needles being taken out any more than you do having them put in. I end up each session with a real sense of comfort and peace.*
>
> Married woman, 48

In theory, the thin acupuncture needles actually stimulate certain nerves that in turn cause the brain to produce *endorphins*—the natural morphinelike substances that produce what is known as the "runner's high." Depending on your complaint, several acupuncture sessions may be necessary to reverse the situation.

Although Chinese medicine has been around for thousands

of years, its growth has been influenced by politics and new discoveries in Western medicine. For example, during the Communist Revolution, Chairman Mao realized there were only 30,000 Western-trained doctors to treat a population of 1 billion, whereas there were many more practitioners trained in classical Chinese medicine. As part of the Communist takeover, Mao promoted the use of Chinese medicine by developing a Boy Scout handbook–type primer called the *Barefoot Manual,* which was used extensively throughout China, especially in remote mountain villages. This resurgence of the practice of Chinese medicine over the past century, coupled with the "rediscovery" of acupuncture's ability to alleviate pain, has resulted in its widespread acceptance and popularity.

Your first visit to a doctor practicing Chinese medicine will include an extensive interview encompassing a complete medical history and lifestyle habits. The doctor's approach is again centered on you as an individual as opposed to your "disease," and treatment is then based on specific imbalances perceived by the doctor. Doctors practicing Chinese medicine feel strongly that no two people are alike and each person requires individual remedies. Treatment usually consists of customized Chinese herbal therapy, acupuncture, or a combination of the two.

According to Dr. Jing Nuan Wu, who practices Chinese herbal medicine and acupuncture in Washington, DC, Chinese medicine can be very effective for women with menopausal indicators like hot flashes, mood swings, and vaginal discomfort. Often the level of success with Chinese herbs and acupuncture is contingent on the individual and other factors such as diet, exercise, and smoking. However, it is possible to manipulate hormonal balance through acupuncture and also impact energy flow, which can cause fatigue and moodiness during menopause.

As effective as Chinese medicine has proven to be over the centuries, its techniques in certain areas, such as fighting infections with antibiotics, are surpassed by Western medicine. A good Chinese doctor will be the first to tell you so and will make appropriate recommendations.

As committed as I am to Chinese medicine, there are times when it just isn't appropriate. When my son had his little finger smashed in a printing press in the art room at school, he needed to take antibiotics to prevent infection. That's why we have modern medicine. But there are so many instances when we can take care of ourselves in other ways if we choose to.

Married mother, 52

Although Chinese medicine was not developed under the careful scrutiny of a regulatory agency such as the FDA, the extensive documentation of thousands of years of practice often go beyond the testing required to introduce a new drug to the market. Nevertheless, it is often difficult for Americans who rely on FDA-approved prescription medication to make the leap to the Chinese medical philosophy. Based on the comments of a wide sampling of American women, it is an alternative worth trying. However, the same caution for homeopathic remedies also holds true for Chinese medicine. Although you may have immediate relief from various midlife complaints, it is unclear whether Chinese medicine provides long-term protection from conditions like osteoporosis. Again, it is important to continue regular monitoring of your bone density and lipid profiles.

Alternative Remedies

Because most of us are conditioned by the drug-oriented techniques of modern medicine, we often believe "strong medicine" is necessary to treat what ails us. As Janine O'Leary Cobb, founder and editor of the menopause newsletter *A Friend Indeed*, points out, "When visiting a doctor, patients often don't feel like they have been properly treated until they're 'awarded' a prescription for their complaint."

The irony is that we have the power to control many aspects of our health by carefully monitoring our diet and exercise regimens. You can have an enormous impact just by paying close attention to your body—what you feed it and how you keep it in shape. This is especially true as you get older and is discussed in detail in the next chapter. To whet your appetite, the following section outlines some of the effects of nutrition and exercise on specific menopausal signs and what you can do as an alternative form of treatment to alleviate those signs.

Nutrition and Exercise
It is almost impossible to create an image that accurately depicts the complexity of the human body and its chemical interactions. The three witches from *Macbeth* stirring eye of newt and toe of frog in their cauldron, however, is a good example of the careful measuring and mixing of just the right ingredients necessary to come up with the perfect potion.

Your body is a highly tuned, sophisticated machine that needs to be kept in balance for peak performance. Too much of one element or not enough of another is all it takes to throw your delicately balanced system out of whack. You probably do not even notice when this balance is only slightly off center, but during the menopausal years, you become more aware of your body as it changes. This can work to your advantage if you pay attention to what is happening and monitor your food and exercise habits.

No two bodies are alike, but overall nutritional and exercise needs are more or less the same. The following parameters for dealing with certain menopausal symptoms are applicable to most women.

HOT FLASH TRIGGERS

Food: Sugar; caffeine; spicy food; garlic; ginger; onions; cayenne; highly acidic foods such as oranges, grapefruits, tomatoes, and berries; hot drinks; and alcohol.
Exercise and conditioning: Exercising in extreme heat, hot baths, and saunas.

HOT FLASH HELPERS

Exercise: Moderate and regular.

Once you see it written on a piece of paper, it is logical that certain foods and environmental factors might contribute to hot flashes. This woman kept track of her habits and was able to identify just what set her off.

I do know that certain things trigger my hot flashes. I've given up wine, unless it's an incredibly good bottle. Drinking wine definitely triggered a flash or two. And stress. Any time I was very angry or upset, I could feel a flash coming on.

Married mother, 46

Depending on the amount and frequency of your sugar indulgence, you can suffer from a roller coaster effect of temperature highs and lows. Instant energy food, sugar rushes into your system and gives it a boost, which also increases your body temperature. It is similar in effect to eating some spicy Mexican food or a hot chili pepper. Caffeine also causes your heart to beat faster, which results in more heat generation. Hot drinks make you hot, and alcohol is just another form of sugar racing through your system. You also heat your body up with a steamy bath or luxurious sauna. The result? More heat. So turn it off yourself and avoid these triggers as much as possible. Every little bit helps.

You can also cope by paying attention to body conditioning and environmental factors. Although exercise as a deterrent to hot flashes has received only slight attention by the scientific community, women who exercise regularly tend to have fewer and less severe hot flashes. A half-hour walk four times a week is worth the effort to stave off some heated evenings.

Dr. Fredi Kronenberg of Columbia University in New York recently completed a study on air temperature and hot flashes. "We looked at the effects of putting women in warm rooms versus cool rooms for eight-hour periods of time and measured the change in the intensity and frequency of hot flashes. It turns out that air temperature has a dramatic effect." Simple as it may sound, Dr. Kronenberg recommends sleeping in a cool room to handle hot flashes that wake you up at night.

Trying to keep cool naturally is great, but if all else fails, you may want to resort to some artificial cooling as this desperate woman was forced to do on a shopping trip to the grocery store.

It was a very hot summer day and I was with my mother in the supermarket. All of a sudden I got this hot flash. Clearly the air-conditioning wasn't having any effect, and for sure it would be worse if I went back outside. Well, they had this huge vertical ice-cream freezer in the next aisle. No one was around, but I said out loud, "Oh, no, the chocolate is way in the back," and I climbed in. I just needed to feel that there was something cold on my face. Wouldn't you know it, my mother rolled the wagon by just then, got a quick picture of what I was doing, and burst out laughing. It was funny, but it worked.

Single mother, 46

OSTEOPOROSIS TRIGGERS

Food: Sugar, protein, caffeine, alcohol, and soda.
Exercise: Sedentary lifestyle.

BONE-BUILDING HELPERS

Food: Calcium-rich substances such as dairy products, nuts, leafy greens, broccoli, rhubarb, salmon, and sardines.
Exercise: Specific weight-bearing activity such as walking, jogging, aerobics, and tennis.

Although the benefits of nutrition and exercise in the prevention of osteoporosis are described in Chapter 3, it is important to emphasize that you have some control over the calcium level in your body. By staying away from certain food that leaches calcium from your bones or inhibits the absorption of new calcium, you are on the right track. Increased calcium intake plus exercise to maintain and build bone mass will make a significant impact on decreasing your odds of developing osteoporosis.

Not in favor of hormone replacement therapy, this woman

has made a conscious effort to stave off osteoporosis with all of the above-mentioned tools.

I've decided not to take estrogen for now, but feel like I want to put a blanket over my head when it comes to the issue of osteoporosis. I try to deal with it by doing weight-bearing exercise, which supposedly makes your bones stronger. I also eat a lot of greens that are high in calcium, like kale, collards, and broccoli. Then I take my little vitamins and do a lot of trusting.

Married woman, 52

MOOD SWING TRIGGERS

Food: Sugar, processed foods, alcohol, and caffeine.

MOOD SWING HELPERS

Food: Several balanced meals eaten throughout the day to maintain blood sugar levels.
Exercise: Twenty minutes of heart-pumping exercise four times a week.

The principle of "whatever goes up must eventually come down" can be applied to the effect certain foods have on your psyche. Many processed foods contain significant amounts of sugar and, when combined with other sweet treats in your diet, can set you up for a real high followed by a mood-crushing low. Alcohol and caffeine act in a similar fashion. Check what you eat and try to stay off the roller coaster.

One natural way to give yourself a lift without any depressing side effects is to get blood moving through your system in the form of exercise. You have heard about the runner's high brought on by the release of endorphins, but you can produce a similar response in your body without being a marathoner. Any aerobic exercise will suffice as long as you get your heart pumping for a good twenty minutes at least four times a week. This is a feel-better guarantee without any addicting side effects.

Vitamins, Minerals, and Other Supplements

In theory, you should be able to get all the nutrients your body needs from daily food intake. In reality, few people eat a well-balanced diet and the food they eat is often processed to such a degree that the essential nutrients are destroyed. Aware of this potential shortfall, many people turn to vitamin and mineral supplements to get what they feel they are missing. If we lived in the year 2050, doctors might be able to do a total body scan, just like in *Star Trek*, to determine the exact balance of existing elements and just what was needed to keep you running in peak condition. Short of that, it makes good sense to consult a physician about taking supplements.

In her book *Menopause Without Medicine* (Alameda, CA: Hunter House, 1992), Linda Ojeda, Ph.D., provides some guidelines about taking supplements. She says women tend to have inadequate intake of both iron and calcium and mentions other conditions that may indicate greater requirements for certain nutrients. According to Dr. Ojeda,

You should consider supplements if you are

- On a diet of less than 1,000 calories per day;
- On a fad diet that restricts a major food group;
- Pregnant, which usually indicates a need for additional iron and folic acid;
- Taking medications (diuretics and some hypertensive drugs deplete potassium; cholestyramine causes poor absorption of fat, vitamins A, B_{12}, D, and the minerals iron and potassium; mineral oil and other laxatives cause a loss of vitamins A and D and the mineral calcium; broad-spectrum antibiotics may decrease vitamin K and some of the B-complex vitamins);
- Diagnosed as having a disease in which diet is a recognized factor: hypertension, heart disease, cancer, kidney disease, ulcers, alcoholism;
- A burn patient, or suffering from a prolonged illness.

Listed below is a broad overview of some of the substances used by complementary physicians in treating women with menopausal complaints. View this as a sampling of potential alternatives, not as a shopping list. If this kind of approach appeals to you, find a doctor who practices complementary medicine so you can have full benefit of the whole body philosophy.

Bioflavonoids

Background	There are more than 400 different types of bioflavonoids, each with a different effect. As a group, they are generally considered very positive for good health. In Japan, where women have few menopausal symptoms and do not even have a word for hot flashes, the average daily consumption of bioflavonoids is 5,000 milligrams daily. In the United States, the average American diet supplies 800–1000 milligrams a day.
Source	Soy products, certain oriental spices, green tea, and citrus fruits (especially the pulp and white of the rind).
Menopausal benefit	Because they have mild estrogenic activity, bioflavonoids provide moderate relief from hot flashes. They also provide some women with relief from anxiety, irritability, and menopause-related mood swings. These same estrogenic qualities may offer some benefit in the prevention of osteoporosis. Medical studies of citrus bioflavonoids indicate their effectiveness with a variety of bleed-

ing problems, including heavy menstrual bleeding.

Dosage   1,000 milligrams, one to three times a day.

Calcium

Background   Calcium is essential to bone health, yet more than 75 percent of women get less than 800 milligrams a day. Worse still, 25 percent of them take in less than 300 milligrams a day, increasing their risk for osteoporosis. Although calcium is readily available in supplement form, it is often difficult to ensure that your body absorbs it. Furthermore, eating large amounts of protein, sugar, soda, and alcohol increases the rate at which your body secretes calcium. A balanced diet, adequate calcium intake, and regular exercise may help in preventing osteoporosis (see Chapter 3).

Source   Dairy products, nuts, leafy greens, broccoli, rhubarb, salmon, and sardines (partial listing).

Menopausal   Before menopause, calcium can help
benefit   increase bone mass density and maintain bone strength. Because women experience a sharp decrease in bone mass for the first five years after menopause, it is important to build bone to its peak density prior to that time. With estrogen replacement, which improves its absorption, calcium has been proven to stem the postmeno-

pausal decrease of bone mass and prevent osteoporosis.

Dosage

1,000–1,500 milligrams of elemental calcium daily for women in their 40s; 1,500 milligrams for women after menopause. To ensure optimal absorption, calcium should be taken with magnesium in a two-to-one ratio (1,500 milligrams calcium/700 milligrams magnesium) and with vitamin D (400 international units) daily.

Evening Primrose Oil

Background

Evening primrose oil is an essential fatty acid, and like all fatty acids, it cannot be manufactured by the body. Fatty acids are critically important in the development of cell membranes and affect the function of the brain, eyes, inner ear, adrenal glands, and reproductive tract. Most adults require 4 teaspoons a day as part of their diet, but menopausal women often have a deficiency and can benefit from 2 or 3 tablespoons a day.

Source

Cold-water high-fat fish such as salmon, tuna, rainbow trout, and mackerel; seed oils such as safflower, sunflower, corn, sesame, and wheat germ; sesame, sunflower, and pumpkin seeds; and wheat germ.

Menopausal
benefit

Well known for its effect on PMS and menstrual cramps, it has also been shown to improve vaginal dryness and promote moister, softer skin. It can postpone the onset of hot flashes for a limited amount of time and seems to enhance the activity of any estrogen that is present in the body. It does not alleviate hot flashes, but it often seems to lessen the severity.

Dosage

Six capsules a day of evening primrose oil, often sold as Efamol. If not available, check ingredients on the label to make certain they include omega-6 fatty acids, cis-linoleic acid, and γ-linolenic acid. Anything labeled "concentrated flaxseed oil" is not the real thing. Because evidence suggests that evening primrose oil has an estrogenic effect, women with a sensitivity to estrogen, especially those with a history of breast cancer or migraine headaches, should use it with caution.

Ginseng

Background

A popular Chinese herb, ginseng root has been used as a medicinal remedy for thousands of years. There are several varieties of this herb, but the one most effective for menopausal complaints is the Chinese or Korean type often called panax ginseng (as opposed to American or Siberian ginseng). Ginseng is basically a stimulant and is usually used to treat any kind of temperature imbalance. Throughout the centuries, it has been claimed to stabilize general bodily systems and counter the effects of aging, weakness, depression, and fatigue due to overexertion.

Source	Chinese and Korean ginseng root.
Menopausal benefit	Because ginseng has estrogenic properties, it is used in combination with other herbs such as dong quai to alleviate hot flashes. Its stimulating effects are also helpful in increasing your energy level and combating fatigue and mild depression.
Dosage	1,000 milligrams daily in two doses. Take on an empty stomach before or between meals. It should not be taken with vitamin C. Ginseng is a stimulant to be used with caution as it can cause insomnia and anxiety.

NOTE: Ginseng's high level of estrogenic activity has been known to cause bleeding in some postmenopausal women and may be an added risk for women with a history of breast cancer.

Magnesium

Background	Magnesium is essential for good bone health and should be taken in conjunction with calcium and vitamin D. It plays a strong role in metabolism and is closely related to energy production. Because modern agricultural techniques often rob food of its natu-

ral nutrients, many people are magnesium deficient. Adequate magnesium levels are also important for the prevention of diabetes and heart disease.

Source	Nuts, whole grains, vegetables, meat, fish, fruit (partial listing).
Menopausal benefit	Magnesium helps in the prevention of osteoporosis by contributing to bone health. It seems to improve the energy of women suffering from fatigue.
Dosage	300–500 milligrams of elemental magnesium daily. Magnesium citrate, magnesium chloride, and magnesium gluconate are recommended because they are more soluble and easily absorbed. Avoid magnesium oxide as it can cause diarrhea.

Natural Progesterone

Background	Like estrogen, progesterone helps build bone tissue and prevent osteoporosis. Natural progesterone may be an alternative to explore in dealing with PMS. (For sources of natural progesterone, see Appendix 2.)
Source	Wild Mexican yams and soybeans.
Menopausal benefit	Progesterone may provide relief from hot flashes, breast tenderness, and migraine headaches. Its role in the prevention of osteoporosis is unknown.
Dosage	Varies, depending on formulation. The dosage is decreased as symptoms lessen and disappear.

Vitamin B Complex

Background

This group of vitamins is important for metabolism and the production of energy from food. New research indicates that several of the B vitamins seem to be effective in enhancing the immune response in the elderly as well as preventing of cervical cancer. Unfortunately, it is easy to become mildly deficient in B vitamins—antibiotics and refined sugar can wipe them out. Synthetic hormones (oral contraceptives and hormone replacement therapy) and even small amounts of alcohol can seriously deplete your reserves of vitamin B_6.

Source

Beans, whole grains, liver, and leafy vegetables (partial listing).

Menopausal benefit

The B vitamins relieve stress. Vitamin B_6, with magnesium, acts as a natural diuretic and can alleviate water retention.

Dosage

One to two tablets daily, depending on the manufacturer's instructions.

Vitamin E

Background

Vitamin E is one of the most well-researched vitamins and is known for its ability to relieve many female complaints. Numerous studies show its effectiveness in improving skin condition, and researchers are documenting its ability to affect cholesterol levels and lower the risk of heart disease. As an antioxidant, it is especially beneficial for city dwellers as it protects against the biological effects of air pollutants. There is also evidence that vitamin E improves immune function in the elderly.

Source

Vegetable oils, nuts, seeds, asparagus, cucumber, haddock, and brown rice (partial listing).

Menopausal benefit

Vitamin E offers some relief from hot flashes, but this effect may take from two to six weeks; helps improve vaginal dryness, especially if applied directly to the vaginal tissue; and decreases breast tenderness caused by PMS.

Dosage

From 400 to 1,200 international units daily, but doses over 600 international units should be taken under medical supervision. Vitamin E should be taken with the mineral selenium (50 micrograms), as the two substances work synergistically.

Vitamins and minerals can be very effective in dealing with menopausal signs. Determined to make them work for her, this woman did some serious research and was rewarded by relief from some pretty severe hot flashes.

I had extreme hot flashes, many a day, and woke up in the middle of the night sopping wet, with terrible sleep disturbances. I was edgy, irritable, and weepy most of the time. With the help of some books on natural remedies, I started treating myself with vitamins, herbs, and minerals. The thing that helped me most with hot flashes and sleeping poorly was taking vitamin E. But it took a while before I figured how much I needed. I started with 200 international units and built up to 1,000 over a six-week period. That finally turned things around for me. It also felt good to take responsibility for my own body.

Married woman, 49

Meditation

Greatly underestimated in Western society, meditation is a well-known alternative treatment for many ailments. So many bodily malfunctions are exacerbated by stress and worry, it is no wonder that meditation is helpful for a wide variety of ills. With the advent of the Lamaze birthing method, many women have already been exposed to a form of meditation through focused breathing and inner concentration. Relying on her experience with meditation, this woman applied it to controlling her hot flashes, and it worked.

I've been meditating off and on for close to twenty years. I found the only thing that would help with my hot flashes was just to be conscious of breathing and focus on relaxing and getting as centered as I could. I started to watch the foods that I ate—I like spicy food and that's not a good thing. I changed the way I dressed and my sleeping habits as well. I used to love my flannel nightgown— now I sleep in a T-shirt. I also keep the window open at night. I made as many alterations as I could. And then I went back to my centered breathing as often as possible. All of it has helped a lot.

Married woman, 51

Menopausal Signs and Solutions

You now have a broad overview of some of the alternatives available to you for treating menopausal signs. The following is a compendium of what you have just read plus herbal remedies found to be effective. Although most herbs have been used extensively for hundreds of years, it is still wise to check the effect of each herb individually by consulting an herbal guide or an appropriate health professional. Also remember, one of your first lines of offense is diet and exercise. Make sure you are eating properly and vigorously moving your muscles several times a week before trying other options.

Breast tenderness	*Vitamins, minerals, supplements:* Vitamin B_6 plus magnesium and vitamin E plus selenium.
Dry skin	*Vitamins, minerals, supplements:* Evening primrose oil and vitamin E plus selenium.
Fatigue, depression	*Vitamins, minerals, supplements:* Vitamin E plus selenium and magnesium. *Herbs:* Blessed thistle, cayenne pepper, dandelion root, ginger, ginseng (panax), and oat straw.
Headaches	*Vitamins, minerals, supplements:* Natural progesterone.
Hot flashes	*Vitamins, minerals, supplements:* Bioflavonoids, evening primrose oil, natural progesterone, and vitamin E plus selenium. *Herbs:* Black cohosh, blue cohosh, dong quai, false unicorn root, fennel, ginseng (panax), red clover, sarsaparilla, unicorn root, and wild yam root.
Insomnia	*Herbs:* Chamomile tea and valerian tea.
Menstrual cramps	*Vitamins, minerals, supplements:* Evening primrose oil.
Mood swings, anxiety, irritability	*Vitamins, minerals, supplements:* Bioflavonoids, vitamin B complex, and vitamin B_6.

| | Herbs: Catnip, hops, passionflower, and peppermint. |
| Osteoporosis prevention | Vitamins, minerals, supplements: Calcium plus magnesium, vitamin C, and vitamin D. Herbs: Comfrey and red raspberry leaf. |

As a final suggestion, you might also want to consider an optimal nutritional supplementation program recommended by Dr. Susan Lark, director of the PMS and Menopause Self-Help Center in San Jose, California, in her book, *The Menopause Self-Help Book* (Berkeley, CA: Celestial Arts, 1990). According to Dr. Lark, "Women with mild to moderate menopause symptoms can use this formula at half strength; women with severe symptoms should use the full strength."

β-Carotene (vitamin A precursor)	5,000 IU
Vitamin A	5,000 IU
Vitamin D	400 IU
Vitamin E	800 IU
Vitamin C	1,000 mg
Bioflavonoids	800 mg
Rutin	200 mg
Vitamin B_1	50 mg
Vitamin B_2	50 mg
Niacin (as niacinamide)	50 mg
Vitamin B_6	30 mg
Vitamin B_{12}	50 μg
Folic acid	400 μg
Biotin	200 μg
Pantothenic acid	50 mg
Choline	50 mg
Inositol	50 mg
para-Aminobenzoic acid	50 mg

Calcium	1,200 mg
Magnesium	320 mg
Iodine	150 μg
Iron	27 mg
Copper	2 mg
Zinc	15 mg
Manganese	10 mg
Potassium	100 mg
Selenium	25 mg
Chromium	100 μg
Bromelain	100 mg
Papain	65 mg
Boron	3 mg

Checking Credentials

For women considering alternative approaches to standard medical care, the choice often revolves around the practitioner's credibility and expertise. Does the practitioner have the ability to listen, thoroughly explain the available treatments, and project credible results? What about education, training, and certification? Is the practitioner's approach and philosophy appealing and understandable?

Alternative does not imply a lower standard. You may not be familiar with the different forms of available treatment, but you should still insist on the same high level of care you would with a more traditional physician. The practice of medicine in the United States is defined as the diagnosis and treatment or cure of a physical condition. Anyone who practices medicine by making a diagnosis or attempting to affect a cure must be licensed. That is the law. Do not mistake enthusiasm for scientific rigor and expertise (see Chapter 10, "How to Get Good Treatment"). Once you are over that hurdle, it is easier to evaluate which alternatives suit you best.

Listed below are the licensure and certification requirements for practitioners of various forms of alternative medicine. If you are uncomfortable checking credentials in person, call ahead and get the information you need from the doctor's office.

- *Complementary medicine* is practiced by licensed medical doctors in all fifty states. There is no organization or association specifically geared toward complementary medicine as there is in Europe. As practiced in this country, complementary medicine is more descriptive than it is a specific school of practice.
- *Acupuncture* is regulated on a state-by-state basis, with differing licensure requirements. If you want verification or a recommendation, the best strategy is to contact your state office of professions to find out which health care professionals are licensed or certified.
- *Homeopathy* in the United States is practiced by licensed physicians, osteopaths, naturopathic physicians, acupuncturists, family nurse practitioners, and physician assistants. Additionally, many lay homeopaths are excellent practitioners. Currently, only Arizona, Connecticut, and Nevada have special licensure for homeopaths.

In his book *Discovering Homeopathy* (Berkeley, CA: North Atlantic Books, 1991), homeopathy advocate Dana Ullman offers some specific guidelines to determine if a homeopathic practitioner is up to par.

1. Find out how much time the practitioner spends with patients. The first visit should be at least one hour, and follow-ups should generally be about twenty or thirty minutes. Less than that may mean that the practitioner does not spend enough time individualizing the correct medicine for you.
2. Find out if the practitioner uses one or more than one medicine at a time. Although there are different ways to practice homeopathy, most experienced practitioners prescribe only one medicine at a time. Good homeopaths

prescribe one medicine for the totality of the person's symptoms and do not usually prescribe one medicine for one disease, a second for another, and so on. There are, however, exceptions to this rule. If you hear that numerous people have received good treatment from a practitioner who uses many medicines, this practitioner may be particularly good with this less traditional approach to homeopathy.

3. Does the practitioner ask you about the totality of your physical, emotional, and mental symptoms? If the practitioner does not ask about your psychological state in reasonable detail, or if he or she focuses entirely on your psychological state, seek a practitioner who is interested in the totality of who you are.

For additional information on how to find a good practitioner, see Appendix 2, page 366.

Covering the Cost

Until some brilliant politician, or more likely a magician, comes up with a comprehensive national health care plan, you will have to either pay directly or rely on insurance companies to cover medical costs. As you have probably discovered, not all medical expenses are covered by insurance, Medicare, or Medicaid. This is especially true when dealing with nontraditional forms of medical care.

Monica Miller, a national health care advocate and currently director of the People's Consortium for Medical Freedom, gives a clear picture of the insurance situation.

Insurance companies insure the unforseeable, the catastrophic accident, that which cannot be anticipated. Yet the philosophy of most alternative therapies revolves around prevention. And until either side gives a little, coverage for most alternative treatment is not in the offing. However, because a good portion of alternative therapy is also used in the treatment of osteoporosis, acute infection, and many other ailments that do not fall into the preventive category, this is an area of ongoing debate.

Specifically, most insurance companies do not cover homeopathy. Some policies cover the cost of acupuncture treatments—typically for anesthesia purposes—but Medicare and Medicaid do not. Finally, alternative therapy prescribed by a complementary medicine physician may or may not be covered depending on how the insurance form is filled out and who is processing the claim.

So before you throw up your hands in frustration, make an assessment about the efficacy of alternative treatment and the preventive philosophy it encompasses. Over the long run, you just might come out ahead both physically and financially.

Chapter Six

Nutrition and Exercise

If you don't take care of your body, you won't have anyplace to live.

—Bumper sticker, 1991

Your Body, Your Palace

Another book with the requisite chapter on diet and exercise? Hardly. Paying attention to the condition of your body is no longer optional once you pass the age of 35. By the time you reach menopause, you must get serious about food and exercise if you want to live the next thirty years in decent shape. *The Bionic Woman* was merely a television series. In real life, this is the only body you have. You must do something to make sure it continues to run in good working order. In the next few pages you will learn about body basics, techniques to assess your physical condition, and strategies to make change less difficult.

A Lifetime Investment
Menopause does not make you fall apart or turn you into a shriveled old woman. Those myths have all been debunked. You will not be able to blame whatever ails you as you get older on this natural phenomenon. Unless you take steps to preserve your body after menopause, however, you will increase your chances of developing osteoporosis and heart disease and, at the same

time, decrease your chances of living a long, healthy, happy, productive life.

No matter what shape you are in right now, you can make changes in your lifestyle and improve the condition of your body. Although most of us started out in good working order, many now have bodies that could use some help. Maybe you feel a little heavy in the thighs, have an extra roll hugging your middle, or get winded from a vigorous walk around the block. Or worse, you lack the energy to play with your kids, are depressed about being overweight, or have surrendered yourself to a sedentary existence. You do not have to spend the next thirty years bemoaning the aging process and feeling sorry for yourself. There is still time to take charge, make some changes, and enjoy life in great physical shape.

Having a weight problem is no fun, and this woman was determined to deal with it earlier in life:

> *I was very overweight when I was 34, a size 16, and went on a rigorous diet. Even though I was bright and my well-rounded figure was passable (this was before the advent of X-ray women), I just thought I was missing something . . . the ability to wear pretty clothes, the freedom to climb a flight of stairs without keeling over, the attention of people when I walked into a room—a sense of liking myself. I managed to get myself down to a size 10 or 8, have maintained that, and feel like I'm in a better position to deal with menopause and middle age.*
>
> Single woman, 50

If you still need motivation, turn back to the earlier part of this book and skim the pages to see the positive impact a well-tuned body can have on mood, attitude, and your risk for osteoporosis and heart disease.

Now is the time to invest in your future. Think of the power you have to control what you eat and how you exercise. You do not need permission or approval from anyone and you are completely in charge. Even if you only incorporate a few of the following ideas into your daily routine, you will still come out ahead. Try to take it one step at a time and do not get discouraged. Like all good investments, your efforts to shape up will pay off in the end.

Nutrition

Eating: One of Life's Greatest Pleasures

Next to sex, there is probably no greater enjoyment than eating. Besides the pleasure you gain from the variety, smell, taste, and sight of food, you also get to partake three times a day. Yum, yum. In order to get the most out of eating, however, you need to know how to do it correctly and without guilt. This is no easy task, especially with paper-thin models supposedly representing the ideal image of today's woman.

Here are a few things you can do to eat to your heart's content—the right way.

Become Educated About Food. You do not need a degree in nutrition to figure out what you should eat on a daily basis. There are plenty of excellent books available (see Appendix 2, "Resources"), and with a little application, you can become quite knowledgeable about what you eat and the effect it will have on your body. Learn which foods are good for you and identify the ones you like to eat. Make sure you also single out foods that may be harmful to your health over the long term.

Just as important is familiarity with your own eating habits. Forget denial and be honest about what foods you like, when you prefer to eat them, and how much you actually consume. You need to understand your preferences and passions so that you can make sure to accommodate them as you make changes.

Identify Bad Habits. You know when you misbehave—own up to it. Do you constantly snack between meals? What about diving for the bread basket when you eat out? Do you watch Jay Leno or David Letterman with food in your hand? How often do you finish up what your partner has left behind? These kinds of questions are not meant to make you feel guilty, but to help you recognize some of the bad habits you may have picked up over the years. You will not be able to change them until you see them for what they are.

It is easy to blame someone or something else for undesirable results, but this woman took a good look at what was really going on, assumed some personal responsibility, and worked on her weight problem.

> *Since menopause, the weight goes on too fast and takes too long to lose. At the time of my menopause, I put on 15 to 20 pounds, almost suddenly. But when I think back and am honest about my passion for chocolate . . . I just think I gave in. I finally lost the pounds and manage to control my weight now, but it's a real struggle.*
>
> *Single woman, 62*

Develop a Commitment to Change. Now that you know what you should eat and understand your personal strengths and weaknesses when it comes to food, it is time to be clear about why you want to make changes. Ideally, you have acknowledged the effects of the natural aging process after menopause and have strong feelings about staying clear of heart disease and osteoporosis. Perhaps you want to wear a size 10 again or feel comfortable at the beach. In any case, you want to look and feel good and are willing to do what it takes to get there. The next step is to make that commitment with religious fervor. You will need it to help you resist temptation, which usually rears its ugly head in the form of potato chips, luscious chocolate, or real ice cream. Make a commitment, not a New Year's resolution, and maintain it for the rest of your healthy life.

In fact, some women do get passionate about making changes at midlife. This busy woman decided it was now or never and set to work toward improving her body with real gusto.

> *I started a diet and exercise program this summer, because on approaching 50, I wanted to be as strong as I could and in a*

position to really enjoy the next stage of my life. I believe that one of the benefits of turning 50 is that you can enjoy doing the things you've been working so hard to prepare for all your life. If you haven't gotten yourself together by then, it's almost too late. From 50 on, you live on what you've built up to that point. So I decided that it was time to get organized and get this body in shape.

Married woman, 49

Make Good Eating Part of Your Daily Life. Easier said than done, this is probably the most difficult part of the task. With today's frenetic pace, reliance on convenience food has reached a new high. It is much easier to reach for a package of precooked goodies than it is to cook from scratch. Most of us do it to save time that can be better spent. So how do you manage to eat properly without devoting all your time to it?

Commitment. Eating properly must assume a higher priority on your daily list of things to be done. You then have a choice: Either learn enough about good food and how to prepare it quickly or block out more time to do it right. The key is to be able to eat the right things without a lot of fuss and bother. You may have to spend more time in the beginning to figure things out—new food to buy, quick ways to cook real food, healthy snacks to have on hand—but it will quickly become part of your new routine.

Be Realistic. The last thing you want to do is fail to take good care of your body. So set realistic goals. After all these years, you probably will not be able to change how you eat overnight. Make it a gradual process and give yourself credit as you go along. Set small interim goals to be sure you make them, all the time keeping your long-term objective in mind. It will not be easy, but the payoff is enormous. Give your body the home it deserves.

What Eating Right Really Means

According to the January 1992 issue of the *Diet & Nutrition Letter*, published by Tufts University, the essence of a balanced diet can be summed up in nine words:

1. more
2. plant
3. foods,
4. fewer
5. animal
6. foods,
7. and
8. more
9. exercise

There is nothing mysterious about it. In the end, eating right is really a balancing act. Imagine yourself on a tightrope, sleekly dressed in a unitard with a long balance pole in your hands. On one end of the pole are foods your body thrives on, like fruits, vegetables, bread, pasta, cereal, low-fat yogurt, and skim milk. On the other are foods you need to be careful about eating, such as meat, chicken, fish, eggs, oil, butter, cheese, nuts, and sweets. The object is to be able to eat what you enjoy and still maintain the balance.

A solid understanding of food is the key to balanced eating. If you increase your knowledge about nutrition, you will be able to expand the choices of foods to pick from and be in total control of what you eat. There is no such thing as good food or bad food. Once you learn how to balance your eating habits, you can usually have some of everything as long as you manage to stay on the tightrope. You will know when it is all right to indulge in a big steak or fudge brownie and when you need to hold back in order to stay in balance. Unfortunately, you will have to deal with temptation, but clear vision and commitment will be an enormous help.

Another important aspect of the balancing act is taste. Unless you come up with an eating plan that tastes good, you will find the balance incredibly difficult to maintain. Every meal you eat must have something you enjoy and all of it should taste terrific. The following sections will show you how to have your cake and eat it, too.

The Gang of Four

Nothing was more boring in grade school than listening to your teacher discuss the four basic food groups: meat, dairy products, grains, and fruits and vegetables. Who cared? After all, your mother made the meals, and it was her responsibility to make sure you ate right. When you became a teenager and had your first chance to make food choices, they often ranged from rebellious to outrageous. Since then, you reached a certain level of moderation and now probably eat from those famous food groups in one way or another.

However, things have changed since the government published its original gang of four recommendations in 1956. There is new thinking about the effects of food on long-term health—some of it hotly debated—and it is all over the map. Still, experts all agree on one issue: Less fat is better. Here are examples of some of the most publicized new nutritional approaches.

- *Revised basic four food groups, currently referred to as the "eating right pyramid,"* is the brainchild of the United States Department of Agriculture (USDA). The pyramid represents a serious departure from previous government recommendations and is in step with current scientific thinking about food and health. At the top, indicating small quantities for daily consumption, are fats, oils, sweets, and dairy and animal products. The broad-based bottom, indicating more numerous daily portions, contains vegetables, fruits, bread, cereal, rice, grains, and pasta. In accordance with American Heart Association guidelines, the USDA recommends a *total* daily fat intake of less than 30 percent of total calories. Finally published in 1992, the pyramid was delayed in response to an uproar by cattle ranchers and the meat industry. The USDA had to deal with two potentially conflicting mandates: to issue nutrition guidelines and promote agriculture at the same time. Ethical minds prevailed, and the new pyramid is truly a model for healthier eating.

fats
oils
sweets (use sparingly)
milk, yogurt, cheese, eggs, nuts,
meat, poultry, fish, dry beans (2–3 servings)
vegetables (3–5 servings) and fruits (2–4 servings)
bread, cereal, rice, grains, and pasta (6–11 servings)

- *The new four food groups*, as proposed by the Physicians Committee for Responsible Medicine, eliminate both dairy and animal products from the mix. According to the committee's director, Dr. Neal Barnard of the Institute for Disease Prevention at George Washington University, most changes to the American diet have been cosmetic. For example, when told to cut down on meat, people increased their intake of fish and chicken. Dr. Barnard feels the majority of people just do not take dietary health warnings seriously and instead accept heart attacks, cancer, and stroke as normal events of later life.

  Although current thinking is to cut down on meat and whole-milk dairy products because they are so high in saturated fat, this organization's radical approach gets rid of them entirely and reorganizes the four groups to include

  Whole grains.
  Vegetables.
  Legumes (beans).
  Fruits.

  Their hearts are in the right place, but it is unlikely Americans are ready to take such drastic action. The group has also been criticized for its misleading name—only 6 percent of its members are physicians.

- *The Cholesterol–Saturated Fat Index* (CSI) is the creation of Dr. William Connor and his wife, Sonja, and represents the first attempt to rank food according to its effect on health risk. In their book, *The New American Diet System* (New York: Simon & Schuster, 1991), the Connors assign a CSI number to each food that reflects its potential to create conditions that contribute to heart attacks and strokes. Using extensive charts and tables listing CSIs for almost any food you can think of, including fast food, you can eat from all food groups providing you do not exceed a preassigned total daily CSI consumption. This is an efficient way to look at all fats combined and assess their damage to your body. Divided into three phases, the New American Diet System gives you time to make changes in the way you eat; overall, it recommends a fat intake of 20 to 25 percent of *total* daily calories. The Connors are lobbying heavily for universal CSI acceptance as a measurement tool and would like it to appear on all package labels to make choices clearer for the consumer.

- *Dr. Dean Ornish's Heart Disease Reversal and Prevention Diets* represent yet another approach to nutrition. Director of the Preventive Medicine Research Institute at the University of California at San Francisco, Dr. Ornish says his prevention diet is for anyone whose ratio of total cholesterol to HDL is more than 3.0 (see Chapter 3, "Postmenopause"). He believes a cholesterol level that will prevent you from having heart disease is around 150 or less. If you are lucky enough to fall into that group, you can continue to eat the way you always do. Unfortunately, the average cholesterol level in the United States is between 240 and 280 and the average American eventually has heart disease. If your ratio is more than 3.0, some changes to your diet are in order. Dr. Ornish's Prevention Diet recommends reducing your *total* fat intake to less than 20 percent of total daily calories.

  If you already have heart disease, Dr. Ornish's Reversal Diet is more drastic and allows a *total* fat intake of less than 10 percent of total daily calories. Because of the high level of fat in animal and some dairy products, you will automatically become almost vegetarian in order to achieve this goal. However, if you have heart disease, learning to eat differently is a small price to pay for improved health.

Although experts may not agree on the details, it is clear they are all heading in the same direction. Less saturated fat, less polyunsaturated fat, less monosaturated fat, less hydrogenated fat. Less fat. Period.

The Big Fat Question

Just when you thought you had everything under control with your knowledge of food and its caloric content, you suddenly get hit with the issue of dietary fat—the latest enemy in your war against unhealthy eating. Sometimes it feels as though a conspiracy is afoot to set up new obstacles: more things to learn, confusing grams to count, and new demons to fight. Fortunately, the latest discoveries on the effect of dietary fat on your weight and overall general health will help you win the battle. That is, once you figure out what it all means.

Despite their differences, the experts all agree Americans must cut down on their daily fat intake in order to survive. Gone are the days of thick, juicy steaks and baked potatoes with butter and sour cream, followed by rich chocolate cake. What is often up for grabs is just how much dietary fat should be allowed each day. From the previous section, you can see the enormous disparity between the American Heart Association's recommendation of less than 30 percent to Dr. Dean Ornish's plea for less than 10 percent. What is the right answer? And how on earth are you supposed to keep track of grams of fat from meal to meal?

To get some perspective on the issue, take a look at the following statistics:

- Eating the current American diet, most people get about 40 percent of their calories from fat, 14 percent of which are from saturated or hardened fat.
- Only 15 percent of American women meet the American Heart Association's recommendation to get no more than 30 percent of their calories from fat.

- Scientific evidence shows a sharp drop in breast and colon cancer rates among people with fat intake less than 20 percent of total daily calories.
- In Japan, which has about half the population of the United States, fat intake is less than 10 percent of total daily calories, and there are 8,000 to 10,000 deaths a year from breast cancer as opposed to 45,000 deaths in the United States.

Why is fat bad for you? Dr. Ornish states the case against fat powerfully in five clear points.

1. Each gram of fat that you eat has over twice as many calories as each gram of protein.
2. Those fat calories are harder to burn off than the same amount of calories from carbohydrates.
3. Dietary fat is easily converted into body fat, whereas very little of the complex carbohydrates in your diet is converted into body fat.
4. Saturated fat increases your blood cholesterol level.
5. Foods high in saturated fat often are high in cholesterol, too.

Obviously, the less fat you eat, the better off you will be, but it is just as important to be realistic about making changes. With that in mind, you might want to reduce your daily fat intake to 20 to 25 percent of total calories. This will mean eating more plant foods and less animal foods, starting right now.

The Real Skinny on Fat

It is easy to have too much of a good thing and that is exactly what we do with fat in our diet. Your body actually needs about 14 grams of fat a day to function properly, but average consumption is usually over 100 grams. No good comes of the extra fat in our bodies and it is time to understand what it is all about.

Fat is fat is fat. In liquid or solid form, it is still fat. Some kinds of it are less harmful than others, but none of it is good for you. All fat is made up of three different elements in varying proportions:

1. *Saturated fat*, the most damaging of the three, raises your cholesterol level and is the primary fat in most animal products. It is the dominant component of butter, coconut oil, mayonnaise, and that tasty bit around the edges of steak and roast beef. Saturated fat enters your body as fat and stays that way, often clinging to the walls of your arteries or depositing itself in unwanted bulges on your hips, thighs, or stomach.
2. *Monounsaturated fat* is found in both animal and vegetable fats and is considered to have no significant effect on blood cholesterol. Oils like olive, peanut, and canola are high in monounsaturates and are definitely better for you than saturated fats.
3. *Polyunsaturated fat* is similar to monounsaturated fat and is much less harmful than saturated fat. Safflower, corn, sunflower, soy, and cottonseed oils are high in polyunsaturates.

Another fat you might see on food labels is *hydrogenated* or *partially hydrogenated fat* or *oil*. This is usually a mono- or polyunsaturated fat that has been converted to a more saturated fat for longer life on your grocer's shelves. Consider it to be a saturated fat and avoid it.

Last, but not least, is *dietary cholesterol*. This type of fat is usually associated with saturated fats from animal products and is harmful to your health. In addition to cholesterol in dairy products, meat, poultry, fish, and shellfish, high amounts of cholesterol are found in egg yolks, liver, kidneys, sweetbreads, and brains. Package labeling has caused a great deal of confusion with products identified as "low cholesterol" or "cholesterol-free." Yes, many of these products are low in cholesterol, but they are often high in other saturated fats. Do not be misled by advertising. Read the label and look for the total amount of fat.

In a nutshell, the objective is to eat as little fat as possible, avoid saturated fat, and limit your fat intake to mono- and polyunsaturated fats whenever you can.

How to Eat Right

If you still have not done some reading on food and learned the basics of good eating, stop everything and do it right away. This is not an intuitive process; you need some education to get it right. Once you have some knowledge under your belt, you will be ready to customize what you have learned and make it work for you. Now is the time to figure out your requirements, discover new ways of eating, and then personally adopt those changes forever.

Take a Number and Learn to Count. This is the easy part. You know what you weigh now and how many calories you can eat every day without putting on more pounds. If you are still unclear, use the tables in one of the nutrition books listed in Appendix 2, "Resources," to figure this out. Next, assume you opt for a daily fat intake of 25 percent or less of total calories. (Go get your calculator at this point.) To determine what that means in terms of daily allowable fat consumption:

- Calculate 25 percent of your total calories.
- Divide that number by 9 (1 gram of fat = 9 calories).
- The final number is the total number of grams of fat you can consume each day.

For example, if your total daily caloric intake is 1,800, multiply that by 0.25 to determine 25 percent ($1,800 \times 0.25 = 450$), and divide 450 by 9 for your total daily maximum fat intake in grams ($450 \div 9 = 50$). This is your number, your maximum number. Try to get below it.

Keeping in mind your total daily calories and allowable grams of fat, do a quick assessment of where you stand with your current eating habits. For the next three days, keep a log of what you eat and when you do it, including estimated portion size and brand names of prepared foods. Then use the tables in one of your nutrition books, or consult appropriate package labels to record rough guesses of caloric content and grams of fat beside every single food item on your list. If possible, distinguish satu-rated fat from mono- and polyunsaturated, and list cholesterol separately. Do the best job you can, even if you can only come up with approximations.

Then add up the columns for each day so you come out with a total number of daily calories and total number of daily grams of fat. The word *total* is used throughout this chapter because there seems to be quite a bit of confusion about where the rec-ommended fat percentage fits. Twenty-five percent fat intake of calories means the percentage of the total calories of everything you eat in an entire day, not meal by meal. Now compare the total calories and grams of fat to your target numbers. This is reality, and if it is not what you need to stay healthy, you know you can do something about it.

This may not be fun, but you need to know where you stand before you start to make changes. You will probably find the answers interesting and perhaps better than you expected.

The Big Change. This is the hard part. Unless you are a vege-tarian who enjoys low-fat dairy products or someone completely up-to-date on low-fat cooking, you will probably have to make some significant changes in what you eat and how you prepare it. Although change will take some work on your part, the time you spend represents a relatively small investment with a huge pay-off. Here are some ways you can approach making these alter-ations.

Change the way you cook. It is amazing to think back twenty years and look at the way you prepared food. Lots of butter, plenty of cream, rib roasts for company, nuts for snacks. Who ever heard of yogurt? Now take a glance at your shopping cart today and you will see that you have already made progress toward eating a more balanced, low-fat diet. Everyone is doing it to one degree or another. Grocery stores have expanded produce sections, food manufacturers offer products with low-fat and low-salt ingredients, and the media constantly sing the praises of healthy eating in articles filled with low-fat recipes. Even famous chefs like Julia Child and Jacques Pépin have new cookbooks on preparing food quickly and with less fat and calories.

With all that support, a little awareness might be all you need. The following examples will help jump start your brain and get you thinking in the right direction.

- *Recipes.* No one said you must follow a recipe to the letter. When it calls for 2 tablespoons of butter, substitute 1 tablespoon of oil. Instead of using heavy cream as instructed, try defatted chicken broth with perhaps some arrowroot for thickening. Experiment a little and lower your fat intake a lot.

  Even older recipes can be modified once you know what they contain. Inexpensive nutrition supplements to more than fifteen popular cookbooks are available and provide per-serving values for the calories, fat, saturated fat, sodium, cholesterol, carbohydrates, and protein (see Appendix 2, "Resources"). One of the better forward-thinking food magazines, *Eating Well,* also provides a service to readers who have favorite recipes loaded with fat. Send them to the magazine and they will literally doctor them up and send you back an up-to-date healthy version.

- *Prepackaged products.* Make them work for you. When you open a can of chicken broth, take an extra few seconds to spoon the chicken fat off the top; you will never miss it. Do not add the 1 or 2 tablespoons of butter recommended on the package for rice and other prepared food. Leave it out and see how it tastes.

- *Low-fat ingredients.* No, skim milk does not taste the same as whole milk, but it is easy to get used to. After a few weeks, most people who make the switch no longer care for the fat-rich variety. The same can be said for many products labeled "lite" or "low fat," and they are worth trying.

- *Fresh fruits and vegetables.* Simply stated, fresh produce tastes better. If it tastes delicious, you will eat more of it. If you do not know how to cook certain vegetables, instead of being embarrassed, learn how. Try using a microwave oven—it is a boon to the harried cook and makes preparing better-tasting vegetables quick and easy.

Most Americans do not even think of fruit as dessert or a healthy snack, perhaps because the majority of supermarket fruit is unripe. So, buy it ahead of time, leave it out in a beautiful bowl to ripen on the coffee table, and see what happens. Or be creative: Peel a banana, wrap it in plastic, stick it in the freezer for a couple of hours or more, and serve frozen slices as a guiltless dessert.

Researchers at Harvard University recently released data suggesting that women who eat just one daily serving of a vegetable or fruit such as carrots, apricots, green leafy vegetables, or spinach have a 40 percent lower risk of suffering from a stroke and 22 percent lower risk of having a heart attack than women who eat very little of these foods. Furthermore, a glass of orange juice in the morning, a lettuce and tomato salad at noon, an apple and carrots for a snack, and broccoli or another vegetable at dinner would exceed the daily quota of fruits and vegetables recommended by the National Cancer Institute to lessen your risk of cancer. Good food for thought.

Whatever you do, there is no reason for good food to taste bad. Learn how to cook a few things well, and if you use fresh food, you can serve it with little or no fuss at all. Invest in some of the new cookbooks and try one recipe a week. You do not have to turn into a gourmet cook in order to eat well.

Change the way you shop. These days you can get into trouble if you are too busy or too lazy to read a label and rely on package headlines instead. Shopping for groceries with a commitment to healthy eating is a lot like moving to a new city. There are familiar landmarks, but you still have to learn your way around town. It takes time, and after only a few days you might find yourself totally lost, sitting three blocks from home with a map in your hand.

At this point, you probably need to turn your next few expeditions to the supermarket into a kind of field trip. Block out the time and spend at least an hour going up and down the aisles with a calculator, reading glasses, and a notepad rather than a shopping list. Do not even think about buying groceries. Locate your favorite products and read the labels on the competition. No doubt you will find big differences in fat and calorie content from one manufacturer to another. Write them down so that you remember the differences when you get ready to make a new shopping list.

The FDA is currently reviewing new labeling formats that will make all of your shopping easier and more nutritious. The strategy is to develop labeling such that you can see how a particular food stacks up compared with the daily recommended amounts for fat, saturated fat, cholesterol, sodium, carbohydrate, fiber, and protein.

Once the new labeling is in place, it will help you focus on your daily intake limits and constantly educate you about different foods and their nutritional values. Until then, you will have to do this all yourself. As soon as you can identify the new items you need to eat right, shopping will become a breeze again. At first it will take some time to find your way around, but eventually you will be able to buy food with more confidence in what it can do for your body.

A few years ago I was getting quite dumpy. I mean, every year I would add a pound or so, and sure enough, when I turned 50, I was ten pounds heavier than I was at 40. It dawned on me that by the time I reached 60, I would be as big as a house. That was when I learned to read food labels, count fat grams, and change my eating habits. It's a drag, but at least I've kept the scales in line.

Married mother, 55

Maintain the balance. Stay on the tightrope by making sure you eat right every day. If you blow it on one meal, make up for it on the next. It is not realistic to make all of the changes mentioned in this chapter overnight. Pick one or two changes, master them, and move on to the next. View each change as a major progression, and give yourself credit—you are on your way to decades of better health and better living.

Exercise

Acknowledge the Necessity

Being physically fit would be so easy if you could just take a little pill once a day and be in terrific shape for the rest of your life. Alas, science has made great strides in this century but still has not discovered a new way to keep muscles toned, hearts healthy, and bones strong, which means exercise is a do-it-yourself project.

These days, it is not enough to look at your body in a mirror and rely on the presence of bulges and sags for inspiration. A quick inspection of the inside of your arteries or a tour of your bone structure might be what you need for motivation, but it is not really feasible. Instead, a fresh look at some of the statistics could be just the ticket to sell you on exercise:

- *Problem*: Women lose 2 to 3 percent of bone mass each year for the first five years after menopause and may lose 30 percent of their bone mineral by the time they reach 70 years of age.
  Possible solution: Bone-loading exercise done daily or a minimum of three times weekly for thirty minutes will help maintain and in some cases increase bone density.

- *Problem*: One in seven women age 45 to 64 has some form of heart disease, and this increases to one in three once you reach 65; concentrations of blood cholesterol, including LDL, or "bad" cholesterol, increase significantly as a result of menopause, usually within six months of the cessation of menstrual periods.
  Possible solution: Studies show that physical activity raises HDL, or good cholesterol, levels, reducing the risk of heart

disease. Physically active women have significantly higher HDL levels.

- *Problem*: Hot flashes plague 80 percent of women around the time of menopause.
- *Possible solution*: Regular physical exercise has been associated with the diminished frequency and degree of hot flashes.

Other menopause factors that might influence your attitude about exercise include mood swings and a tendency toward weight gain. Psychologists and athletes have known for years that exercise has a direct effect on mood and overall outlook on life. This woman took her doctor's advice and definitely came out ahead of the game.

I've found that diet really seems to affect my moods. So does exercise. At my doctor's suggestion, I cut down on caffeine and sugar, started drinking more water, and got out and walked almost every day. What a difference. Before, when I felt moody, I just wanted to sit in a corner, munch on some chips or chocolate, and be left alone. These days I go out for a walk and feel 100 percent better.

Single woman, 48

Although it has been proven that menopause, in and of itself, does not cause depression, other events at midlife can often bring on the blues. Feelings expressed by this woman are not unusual for women at midlife and her solution is one that should be taken to heart.

There are so many things that happen when you're middle-aged that it's hard to know what's what. Are you feeling depressed because your best friend is losing her husband? Are you down because of the recession? Are you depressed over no longer being able to produce children? The single most important factor that makes the biggest difference when I'm feeling this way is exercise.

My weekly aerobic exercise class makes all the difference in the world.

Married mother, 52

As much as you try to fight it, weight gain is a reality for many midlife women and not just those taking hormone replacement therapy. With aging, your body's metabolism slows and unless you change your eating habits and, more importantly, include exercise in your daily routine, you are bound to put on the pounds. Going on a crash diet, like you may have done as a younger woman, will not be effective. In the long run, you will have to exercise to stay even.

What's happening to my body as I get older is the bloody pits. You have to work harder at staying in shape and if you're not on some kind of regular exercise regimen, you're in real trouble. There was a time when I could drop five pounds like that, without lifting a finger. Now, the only way to lose it and keep your skin from looking like an extra layer of clothes is to exercise.

Married mother, 51

Over and over, studies show that physically active people are healthier and happier than those who lead a sedentary life. And they live longer. Exercise also improves your skin, elevates mood, and burns calories. All in all, the decision to exercise is a no-brainer.

How to Get There from Here

To most people, exercise is just another word for torture. Unless it is disguised as a tennis match, a bicycle ride to the beach, or an evening of dancing, exercise is second only to a visit to the dentist. Today's lifestyle does not naturally include exercise, unless you live on a farm or work outdoors, and instead it must be artificially included in your daily schedule. However, it is possible to enjoy exercise and do it on a regular basis if you follow these suggestions.

Visualize Yourself as Physically Fit. In order to have a clear picture of your exercise goal, the first step is to abandon images of Jane, Cher, and Raquel. Be realistic. Find a reasonable role model, someone who is not a model or a film star and who is committed to physical fitness. Think of yourself in the same good condition and keep that picture in the front of your brain every day.

Sample the Choices. Whether you are in your late 40s or early 60s, you are not too old to participate in a wide variety of physical activities. You have probably tried walking or even running, but what about ice skating, swimming, tennis (no, it is not too late), bicycling at home or on the road, dancing, rowing or canoeing, hiking, badminton, golf (if you walk the course), and cross-country skiing? Spend some time sampling without making a commitment to any single activity. You may discover something you never thought you would enjoy. Just think how easy exercise might be if you actually had a good time.

Exercise almost turned into a political issue for this woman who was bound and determined to get on a bicycle again for a regular workout. Despite the need for some mechanical updating to make her bicycling vision a reality, she clearly used the power of her personality and self-confidence to make it all work out.

> They're definitely building bicycles for the wrong people. I just bought a new one and had a terrible time—the seat was too skinny, the angle was wrong, and the handlebars were ridiculous. I think I went back to the shop about 800 times until they got it right. I made them put on old-fashioned handlebars and make a bunch of other adjustments until I felt I could be comfortable riding for hours. In the end, I gave the man in the shop a piece of my mind and told him, "There are a lot of us older folks around, but we're in good health and very active. So, if you want to have a growing business, you'd better start building bikes for us."
>
> Married mother, 54

Set Yourself Up for Success. This is not a game. Exercise must become an important part of your life in order to do it on a regular basis. This means your choice should accommodate your lifestyle. If you travel a great deal, make arrangements to walk or run while on the road. If you have a busy schedule and live by a calendar, make an appointment every day for your exercise routine—just block out the time like you would for any other engagement. Then reward yourself every time you do it. If everything else in your day is going wrong, you can at least point to the thirty minutes you spent working out as a solid accomplishment.

> *I'm not a jogger, but I do love to walk and try to do it whenever I can. I commute to the office by railroad, so I put in a half mile each day just walking to the station and back. In the evening, if I get a ride, I'll try to walk around the neighborhood. And during the summer, I try to swim just to get some extra exercise.*
>
> *Single woman, 58*

Unfortunately, no matter how compelling the evidence, some women just cannot get it together to exercise on a regular basis. For them exercise is anathema, as voiced by this well-intentioned woman. Nevertheless, as distasteful as it is to her, she does manage to work out from time to time.

> *I don't like to exercise. I have never liked it. I know I'll feel wonderful afterward. But there are times when you are just so tired—the last thing you want to do is work out. I guess I just force myself to go do it. I have to consciously make myself remember to do it, even though I know the payoff is tremendous. It's just not part of who I am. I'm driven to work in my garden, not to go for a three-mile walk.*
>
> *Married woman, 54*

Exercise—A Little Goes a Long Way

The good news is that you do not have to be a world-class athlete to reap the benefits of exercise. Nor do you need to spend vast quantities of time at the gym. What you do need is the knowledge of how much and what kind of exercise works best and a serious commitment to doing it.

At last the experts are in agreement when it comes to the amount of exercise required to maintain good health. Moderation and regularity are the operative words and all it takes is

- Thirty minutes of walking or similar activity once a day, every day, or
- Sixty minutes of walking three times a week.

No fancy equipment, special classes, and expense are necessary. The amount of exercise prescribed above will help to lower your risk of osteoporosis, heart disease, diabetes, and obesity. This is all it takes. Simple, easy, doable. You have just run out of excuses.

After being hounded into submission by her doctor, this woman developed a new attitude about exercise, one that is easier to achieve once you internalize the health benefits of regular exercise.

> *After seeing a doctor about osteoporosis and hearing about exercise for the umpteenth time, I've finally gotten the message. My body has responded well to walking almost every day and I can feel the difference. But the big revelation for me was figuring out that I was the one who was responsible for my body, not my doctor. It's a good feeling to be in control, walk down the street, and not worry anymore about getting enough exercise . . . almost like a sense of freedom.*
>
> Married mother, 59

If you want to count calories as a further incentive, you burn off about 100 calories for every mile you walk briskly or jog. To give you perspective on other activities, each of the following burns about 2,000 calories:

- Walking four miles in one hour, five days a week.
- Running three miles in thirty minutes, six days a week.
- Playing singles tennis for one hour, five days a week.
- Swimming for thirty minutes, six days a week.

- Cross-country skiing for thirty minutes, six days a week.
- Aerobic dancing for forty minutes, five days a week.

There is no reason for regular exercise to be an insurmountable goal. This is something you can control and receive positive benefits from almost immediately. As they say in the ads, just do it.

The Turning Point

Sometimes all it takes is a single event to significantly influence and even change your way of thinking about previously ingrained habits or beliefs. For many women, the dramatic physical changes associated with menopause are all it takes to modify a routine or introduce new behavior patterns. Often a change of venue can be the impetus to trying new things, as this postmenopausal woman discovered after moving to the West Coast.

Exercise is not something I've done all my life, but I took it up in a big way when I moved to California. I met a number of exercise teachers and took yoga and stretching. I've been in an exercise program ever since and learned to play tennis—all of which happened way after I passed menopause. I always thought I was a sedentary person. I'm mentally healthier since I started an exercise routine, and it has a calming effect on my whole personality. It's funny, I'm so much more active than I was in my younger days.
Married mother, 68

This does not imply that you need to make a cross-country move to start an exercise routine. Often, little tidbits in the news are all it takes to get the ball rolling, like one recently published in the *New York Times* that stated that the average American woman is 5'3" tall and weighs 144 pounds. If you weigh in at 135 and still feel complacent about this profile, perhaps some other statistic or bit of medical news will be inspiring.

Menopause is a turning point in a woman's life whether she chooses to acknowledge it or not. With a positive attitude, you can make all the physical change and emotional upheaval work for you, just like this woman plagued by malaise at midlife.

I'm not a high-energy person, and in my late 40s, when I started to go through menopause, I got even less energetic. So I signed up for a diet and exercise program at a local sports club. All you had to do on this program was exercise for twenty minutes, three times a week, with a trainer. Piece of cake, I thought. Wrong—it damned near killed me! I have never been in such pain and agony in my whole life, and there were times when I would stagger home and just fall into bed. After about four weeks of feeling like I was going to die, I got a burst of energy and came alive. I don't know what happened, but I haven't been the same since. They said I lost ten pounds of fat but gained five pounds of muscle. Since then, I've lost more weight and still keep up with a training program. I work out twice a week for twenty minutes, walk for twenty minutes, and that's it. But I have more strength and energy now than I've had in my whole life.

Single mother, 51

The message is clear—you need only to act on it.

Chapter Seven

Sex

After 50, a man's performance is of poor quality, the intervals between are wide, and its satisfactions of no great value to either party. Whereas his great-grandmother is as good as new.

—Mark Twain (1835–1910)

Older women clearly had the sexual advantage in Twain's opinion, and more courageous men today might still agree. So what is the panic all about?

Menopause definitely marks the end of your reproductive ability, but by no means does it herald the end of your sex life. Quite the opposite, in fact. Many postmenopausal women—admittedly after an oftentimes rocky start—report increased desire, no more worries about contraception, and a welcome reprieve from menstrual miseries like excessive bleeding, cramping, and mood swings.

If anything, menopause has added to my sex life. I no longer worry about getting pregnant and that was always a big issue. I'm of a generation that did not go on birth control pills. I used a diaphragm, but like everyone else, I slipped out of the habit every now and then. So menopause has relieved pressure and anxiety about accidental pregnancy. Sure, there are body changes to deal with and I do have to use a lubricant at times.

But menopause has not decreased my performance or desire for sex.

Single woman, 58

As their focus shifts from raising children or climbing the corporate ladder, many women are less stressed and find they have more time than ever to enjoy sex, discover sex anew, or, for some, learn about the joys of sex for the first time. In fact, based on a study of sexual behavior of women in their 60s, Dr. Gloria Bachmann of the Robert Wood Johnson Medical School reports, "Sex is alive and well in older women."

There is no question that women entering menopause today are a breed apart from any other generation of perimenopausal women in history. Not only do we lead active full lives, but we also are decidedly interested in sex. Flower children, Age of Aquarius, free love, and open marriage are just some of the watchwords of our generation. With the advent of the birth control pill, many of us were free from the perils of unwanted pregnancy. We no longer looked at sex as a conjugal obligation and instead discarded the restrictions of sex only after marriage, experimented with several partners (pre-AIDS), and discovered the many pleasures of sex. Sexual interest exists for older women and men, and being menopausal does not mean that you are over the hill.

However, the sexual picture for postmenopausal women is not totally rosy. Two separate studies conducted by Dr. Phillip M. Sarrel, an obstetrician and psychiatrist at Yale University's School of Medicine, showed that sexual problems were extensive in 178 postmenopausal married women in London who were 35 to 62 years of age. Of this group,

- 154 women said they had sexual problems.
- 45 percent reported a loss of sexual drive.
- 10 percent said they had developed an aversion to sex.
- 27 percent said they could no longer reach orgasm.
- 43 percent complained of vaginal pain and dryness.

Only 24 women said they had no sexual problems at all.

As you might expect, the second study showed that men were also affected as they age. Some of them became impotent and lost their ability to reach orgasm. The men also expressed feelings of rejection and anger, a fear of hurting their partners, and concern about their ability to perform sexually.

These bleak statistics can make it difficult to adopt a "you're not getting older, you're just getting better" philosophy. However, that is just what you must do to make it through the transition of menopause and ensure yourself a fulfilling sex life.

When we were in a bad place in our marriage, my husband said, "We don't have sex enough." "No," I said. "The problem is we have a problem. And if we didn't have a problem, we'd have sex."
Married mother, 47

If you experience menopausal sexual problems, the first step to solving them is easy—recognize the changes in your body, pay attention to them, and take action. Noted health author and columnist Jane E. Brody says, "Since 'use it or lose it' seems to be an important component of continued sexual functioning after menopause, it is important not to delay seeking help for sexual problems. Such problems are easier to correct before they become advanced and complicated by emotional reactions."

The second step is to evaluate the problem. Is it related to one of the physical changes of menopause and therefore temporary if properly treated? Or is it part of some larger problem related to your sex life that has existed in one way or another for many years? What about emotional issues related to sex? Have you forgotten that 90 percent of sexual drive is still centered in the brain?

The third step, communication, is the hardest. Once you recognize and understand the nature of your sexual problem, you will have to talk about it with someone—your partner, doctor, sister, friend, or psychologist. For most of us, talking about sex is a daunting prospect. Although women are candid and open in general, when it comes to frank discussion about personal sexual issues, they are often at a loss for words. There are definitely ways to learn how to communicate about sex without dying a million deaths, and they are described later in this chapter. For now, think of communication as the key to unlocking your postmenopausal sexual potential.

Some Perspective on Sexual Response

Even though you have been having sex for years, a review of the basics will help you understand your body as it gets older. Sexual response is specific and a variety of changes occur throughout your body during arousal. When a woman gets excited, the pelvic area fills with blood and the vagina begins to sweat, or lubricate, in anticipation of intercourse. As you become increasingly excited, your clitoris engorges with blood and becomes enlarged, your heart rate increases, and the upper part of your vagina lengthens and expands while the part nearest the vaginal opening becomes firm. During orgasm, a woman experiences rhythmic contractions—from mild to "wow," from just a couple to multiple. After orgasm, a sense of physical relaxation occurs. Finally, during the last phase of sexual response, called *resolution*, women often experience a hypersensitivity in their genital area. This is a time when women can be aroused again and experience additional orgasms, whereas men, especially as they get older, generally cannot.

These female patterns of sexual response remain essentially the same throughout life, but as women age, sexual response slows slightly and becomes a little less intense. It does not disappear. According to gerontologist Dr. Ruth Weg of the University of Southern California, older women take longer to become lubricated and achieve clitoral elevation—it may take a woman in her 40s five minutes as opposed to the fifteen to forty seconds it took in her 20s. Unless a woman has been very sexually active, by the time she turns 50, orgasms will be shorter and uterine contractions will drop from two to three per orgasm to one or two. This is hardly cataclysmic, and having fewer contractions does not necessarily lessen the pleasure. The resolution phase is also shorter in postmenopausal women. Weg says, "If excitation is sufficient, women at any age can be sexually responsive. Genital response is only one measure of the total sexual experience."

Physical Changes at Menopause

Life is always a trade-off. With menopause, you no longer have to contend with the bothersome aspects of reproductive life, but you do have to deal with a new set of body challenges. As your estrogen levels decrease during perimenopause, changes in your vagina, urinary tract, cervix, uterus, and response receptors will become noticeable and have an effect on your sex life. Later in this chapter you will learn what you can do to cope with these changes and keep your sex life in good condition.

Vaginal Changes

The most notable sign of menopause, vaginal changes are second only to hot flashes in causing consternation and frustration. As your estrogen supply diminishes, your vagina begins to shrink in size—both in height and width. It loses its elasticity and becomes thinner, making it easier to bruise and tear. The vaginal lips also become more delicate and are easily irritated. To make matters worse, vaginal lubrication, which is essential for comfortable sex, decreases or slows substantially. Itching and irritation frequently accompany this vaginal dryness. Many midlife women are still not aware of these changes.

> I never knew vaginal dryness was a part of menopause. It wasn't until I went to a conference on midlife health and heard the speaker mention it a few times that I began to put two and two together and was able to account for the pain I'd had on several occasions. Not all of which occurred in the bedroom, I might add. The last couple of times I went for a Pap smear, it was tremendously uncomfortable. I complained during my examination, but

all the doctor said was, "Relax, relax, relax." I'm embarrassed to say that I didn't know what was going on, but I also didn't get much help from my doctor either. Now that I know what's happening to my body, I can at least take steps to turn this painful situation around.

Married mother, 53

With all of these changes, experienced by 25 percent of women only five years after menopause, you can easily imagine the havoc wreaked on your sex life. Intercourse can become painful, penetration difficult to achieve, and bleeding after sex may occur as a result of trauma to the thinning vaginal walls.

These are real physical changes, none of which springs from your imagination. They can be a serious turnoff to sex for women and their partners. However, these changes are often reversible, even after long periods of time. Maintaining a sense of humor also helps, as this woman did when confronted with vaginal dryness.

If vaginal dryness is going to affect my sex life in certain ways, then I'm going to have to learn other avenues. I've bought several books on massage with this in mind. I figured I can give my mate a good massage, let him fall sensually asleep, then, when he wakes up, say, "Wasn't I terrific!"

Single woman, 49

Do not let this get out of hand and spell the end of your sex life, and avoid feeling shame or embarrassment about the situation. Get help right away (see Chapter 2, "What's Going to Happen to Me? . . . Perimenopause").

Cervical and Uterine Changes

Just as the vagina is affected by decreasing estrogen levels, so, too, are the uterus and cervix, which become smaller in size. This may lead to "painful" uterine contractions during and after orgasm for some women. However, your ability to reach orgasm is not related to estrogen levels.

Lessened Response to Stimulation

During this time, you may find that it takes longer to get turned on and respond to sexual stimulation. No, your partner is not losing expertise or even sex appeal. Although the reasons are unclear, menopausal women often have a diminished response to sexual stimulation, especially during the first part of lovemaking. Masters and Johnson, the famous sex researchers, found that after menopause many women experience a delayed reaction of the clitoris to stimulation and less expansion of the vagina during intercourse. If this is combined with discomfort caused by less lubrication, your ability to enjoy sensory stimulation can be greatly diminished. This is not a figment of your imagination.

Men's Physical Changes

> Some older men may say their erections aren't as big as they recall them once being. But then their partner says, "Well, dear, you overestimated them back then, too."
> —Dr. Paul T. Costa, Jr., psychologist,
> National Institute on Aging

While you may bemoan the changes happening to your body during menopause, you are not alone. Men are not immune to the effects of aging physically, emotionally, or sexually. There are two species involved in heterosexual sex, and physical changes in men can have significant impact on lovemaking as both partners get older. However, men undergo a gradual modification of their sexual response rather than the radical hormonal changes women experience during menopause.

I do think that men go through changes as they age. The only reason it's not a big deal is that men's changes are not as visible as women's menopause. But their changes should be acknowledged. If more emphasis was placed on their side of the equation, then perhaps women wouldn't take such a bad rap for their complaints about menopause. These transitions are important for both males and females.

Single mother, 49

Here is the short list of some of men's physical changes:

- Erections come slower.
- A longer time is required to achieve a firm erection, and more direct physical stimulation is often needed.
- The need for orgasm (ejaculation) may decline, although this does not necessarily mean sexual desire wanes. Men just may not feel the need or urge to ejaculate each time.
- The ability to maintain an erection for longer periods of time increases (often a real plus for women).
- Ejaculation may be less forceful; semen will not be expelled with as great pressure as before.
- Erections tend to fade faster after ejaculation.
- The time between erections increases, and by the age of 60, it can take up to twenty-four hours for men to have another erection.

These are not inconsequential changes although it is doubtful that you have ever heard a man talk about them. Many women who are focused on their own changes often misread the altered performance of their aging partners as a lack of sexual interest. This just is not so. Men may get discouraged or embarrassed by their diminished sexual prowess, but their interest usually does not wane. Keep this in mind in bed.

Sex is so much better now than when I was younger. You know, I really think Mother Nature messed up. I mean, we get so out of sync with men as we get older. Men start to slow down and women are raring to go. My husband looks at me sometimes and says, "Where have you been all my life?"

Married mother, 52

The Libido Conundrum

Although most sexual taboos have disappeared, women are still reticent to utter a single word about loss of desire. For some unknown reason, lack of libido is often taken as a personal shortcoming—"There must be something wrong with me"—making it difficult for women to confront and deal with the situation.

Well, brace yourself. Many women experience some decrease in sexual desire by the time they reach 54. This is a normal part of the aging process, and its intensity varies for each individual. Women who have sex infrequently are more likely to experience diminished desire in their 60s; those who are more sexually active will probably not notice any significant change.

I have completely lost my libido and can no longer achieve orgasm. I didn't know what was happening to me until I read a magazine article about it. I remember running in and showing it to my husband and saying, "Look at this, I'm not alone." I feel I'm cheating my husband, and that's not a good situation to be in. He's not handling it well, and I really can't blame him. He's a type A personality, a salesman, and very dynamic. Even though he's one of the tops in his field, when it comes to sex, he likes me to be the initiator. Well, at this point in my life, I just can't. In the beginning, my husband thought it was his fault and that I was no longer attracted to him. We've talked since then, and at this point, I think he finally understands that it's something that I'm going through and not anything he has caused.

Married mother, 56

Although a change in libido usually occurs during your menopausal years, declining estrogen and testosterone levels, in and of themselves, are only partly to blame. Like most emotions, libido is affected by a combination of factors working together: sex hormones, psyche, environment, and your partner, just to name a few. Sexual drive is multifaceted, and variability of a single factor will not necessarily affect its strength.

However, doctors now think that some postmenopausal

women who report loss of libido may have low testosterone levels. Testosterone, a sex hormone like estrogen, is produced by both men and women and is known to drive sexual interest. In women, it is produced by the ovaries (even after menopause to some degree) and the adrenal glands. You can request measurement of your testosterone levels the same way you request your doctor to measure estrogen. This is worth investigating and may be a significant factor influencing your libido. It can be hurtful to you and your partner to blame psychological causes when a decrease in libido may be the result of a hormonal decline.

You May Have an Attitude

Loss of libido at menopause is not a cut-and-dried issue. A lot of it may be the effects of an old wives' tale, having more to do with the traditional female role than with physiological facts. Libido is a lot more complex than merely the sum of your body parts: The mind plays a big role in whether or not you want to have sex.

Even with a contemporary outlook on menopause and aging, many women still retain the image of a dried-up old woman in the far recesses of their brains. That haglike creature of your imagination certainly did not just tumble out of a love nest ready for her next sexual encounter. Why do women still think this way? Is it because there are no role models of menopausal women with sex appeal other than femmes fatales like Elizabeth Taylor, Sophia Loren, and Joan Collins? Or is it because women are afraid to confront a change in their sexual attitude?

Many women lose sexual desire at menopause because that is what they think they are supposed to do. Talk about a self-fulfilling prophecy. In spite of physical evidence to the contrary, they may think their sex appeal has gone down the drain and they are no longer desirable to their partners. Or because they have lost the ability to reproduce, they may think they are no longer really women and certainly not sexual beings.

I think women feel insecure when they see their husbands walk down the street looking at all these sweet young women. It makes women feel uncomfortable, maybe because they feel they can't compete anymore. The funny thing is, you don't have to compete with a younger woman because you have much more to offer in many ways. You just have to learn how to use your strong points to better advantage. Women who go through this kind of thing start to confront issues they haven't dealt with yet. A lot of women have sexual hang-ups they never really had to cope with before because they were able to get by when they were younger. So rather than confront them or do something about it, they often just fall deeper and deeper into the pits.

Married woman, 49

Painful sex due to vaginal problems, or *dyspareunia*, can also have an insidious effect on your libido. Memory of pain and its association with lovemaking can cause women to physically and mentally turn off to any and all sexual stimulation. Even a single uncomfortable encounter can negatively influence your libido. It is essential to nip this physical problem in the bud and get help before it blossoms into an emotional issue.

If you retain even the slightest interest in sex, there is no reason to buy into negative thinking. Menopause can be a catalyst to make things different in bed. View this time with a half-full, as opposed to half-empty, attitude and you will be rewarded with a new kind of closeness with your partner.

My attitude toward sex has definitely changed since menopause. For the first twenty-five years of our marriage, it was fun and enjoyable. And it got more interesting after I stopped having my period. What a wonderful sense of relief to not worry about getting pregnant anymore. But then that excitement seemed to wear off, and sex doesn't seem to be as important as it was. There's no point in being artificial about it and trying to have sex when neither of you is in the mood. Let's face it, you have to find ways to make sex more exciting. And that goes for both partners. Most of all, there has to be a closeness, a very strong relationship with both people caring enough to keep each other happy.

Married mother, 55

Sex? No, Thank You

One of the best-kept secrets of middle age is that some women no longer want sex. Period. Some women welcome menopause as an excuse to discontinue sex—an activity they never really enjoyed. Now that they are "past their prime," they do not have to pretend anymore. This is not a crime or something to feel ashamed about. For these women, sex is just not a be-all-and-end-all experience. They seek and find intimacy and ways of being together with their partners outside of the realm of sexual intercourse, and it works for them.

Some of your best friends may not be very interested in sex, as this woman recently discovered.

> I'm amazed by the number of friends my age who don't like sex, who haven't had a good sexual experience, who still see sex as "Lie on your back, close your eyes, and think of England." Therefore, when they go through menopause, whether it's a result of disease or nature, they view it as a welcome relief. They don't have to have sex anymore because they can now say it hurts. There are lots of women out there who just don't want sex. They probably grew up in an environment where sex was a dirty word. In fact when one of my friends heard I had become menopausal, she gleefully said, "You're lucky, you'll never have to do that again." Totally surprised, I replied, "I enjoy that and have no intention of giving it up." There are lots of women out there who feel just like my friend.
>
> Single woman, 52

This lack of sexual interest was evident in a study of middle-aged women and sexuality reported by Dr. Ellen Cole, sex therapist and coeditor of the journal *Women and Therapy*. In interviews with women questioned about their decreased sexual desire, some of them mourned their current situation, truly enjoyed being sexually active, felt it was an important part of their identity, and wanted it back. Other women said they did not really care about their loss of libido. They viewed this as a stage in their development, a time when they were moving on to other things, relationships were changing, and they were very content.

What is normal anyway? According to Dr. Phyllis Kernoff Mansfield, associate professor of health education and women's studies at Pennsylvania State University, "One of the big mistakes women make is to make judgments about what a 'healthy sex life' means on the basis of what they did as 20- or 30-year-olds. Women automatically assume having low interest in sex is wrong and probably a personality disorder." Sex is a personal issue, and it is up to you to decide what is right, comfortable, and enjoyable.

Getting It Regular

One of the great things about being an adult is that it is all right to have sex, safe sex. One of the most versatile tonics for many menopausal indicators is regular sex. So, for those who enjoy a romp in the hay, this is great news.

What Is Regular?

Masters and Johnson, who coined the phrase "use it or lose it," observed that women who have sex once or twice a week throughout their lives have better and quicker lubrication after menopause. Once or twice a week is all it takes, whether you have intercourse or masturbate. Orgasm is not the issue here; stimulation is what is needed to keep your vagina in good working order.

Menopausal Benefits

In addition to preventing vaginal dryness, regular sex keeps estrogen levels up and increases blood supply to the entire reproductive and urinary area. Even in postmenopausal women, vaginal stimulation seems to increase estrogen levels. It can reduce hot flashes to a mild degree and hold off vaginal atrophy by keeping the vagina—which is, after all, a muscle—in shape. Like any exercise, sex is good for your cardiovascular system and can give your heart a solid workout. As you might expect, desire breeds desire. Regular sex will keep you coming back for more.

Sexual Frequency Factors

Sex is not quite as simple as putting on a pair of shoes, and it is not easy to determine where you might fit in the sexual picture after menopause. Interpersonal, rather than hormonal, factors appear to be the best predictors of which women will remain sexually active into their 60s and beyond. In her research on postmenopausal women, Dr. Bachmann concluded that other factors, such as the availability of a functional partner, cultural and religious attitudes toward sexuality, and chronic illness, are often reported as important determinants of sexual interest, especially in women 50 years and older.

Age. Even with all the benefits of regular sex, studies show sexual frequency tends to decline as people age. A recent study of sexual practices in the United States found that people 50 to 59 had sex an average of forty-six times a year—almost once a week. An older group of 60- to 69-year-olds cut that amount almost in half with sexual activity twenty-three times a year; the oldest group of people over 70 had sex only eight times a year.

However, with the huge number of baby boomers entering middle age, this picture might be improving. In fact, with an increasing awareness of the aging process, communication between middle- and old-agers may increase and perhaps spark some inspiration, much like that experienced by this woman in her late 50s.

> *I think things are changing. Our society is growing older, and we are getting used to seeing people of older ages all around us. I have friends who are in their 80s, who look and act as though they feel they're in their 60s and who have active sex lives. So today, being 60 doesn't seem that old and even turning 80 is not so bad a prospect. I sat next to an 88-year-old woman at a lecture a few nights ago, and she looked fabulous. She's very with it, and when I asked her why she still looked so good, she said, "I have an active sex life." Based on her comments, if I play my cards right, I've got another thirty years of fun ahead of me.*
>
> Single woman, 58

Sexual Satisfaction. According to Dr. Bachmann, sexual satisfaction seems to be another indicator of sexual frequency after menopause. In her study of fifty-nine women in their 60s, Dr. Bachmann found "abstinent women not only reported significantly less sexual satisfaction with current encounters, but over the entire course of their marital relationship they recalled less sexual satisfaction and less comfort in expressing sexual preferences than women who were coitally active. It may be the case that continued interest in sexual activities as one ages is at least partially dependent on having enjoyed satisfactory sexual exchange earlier in life."

Marital Status and Sexual Orientation. Sexual activity can also be influenced by marital status. A study of sexual practices in the United States reported married people had sex an average of sixty-seven times in the past year; divorced and never-married singles an average of fifty-five times; separated people an average of sixty-six times; widows and widowers averaged six times.

However, there is more to the story than statistics. Marital status also affects how women feel about themselves, which, of course, influences their sex lives. For example, in a recent study comparing women at midlife, there was a significant difference between married and single women. Women who were single at midlife reported feeling very good about their body changes and feeling attractive as they got older. Married women, in the same study, said they felt very unattractive as they became middle-aged.

Even though menopausal single women feel more attractive than married women, they often have a harder time finding sexual fulfillment at midlife.

Sex is different now—there's no question about it. Before menopause I knew I could have an orgasm within two minutes. Now I'm not so sure how long it will take, and this is just with masturbation. I've had trouble with vaginal dryness and even though I'm on hormones, I am very scared about having sex with a man again. It feels like I'm a virgin who doesn't know what to do. I look good. I feel good. But I haven't met a man to test my sexuality with. I was at a party recently with about ninety people. Great music, and I was dancing up a storm when all of a sudden I spotted my gynecologist, who is also a friend. He came over, gave me a hug, and said, "I see those hormones are working." I thought to myself, Isn't anything sacred? and replied, "Well, I haven't tested them completely yet, but I'm working on it!"

Single mother, 45

Sexual orientation also seems to be a factor in sexual satisfaction. In a study by Dr. Ellen Cole, lesbians did not report the same kind of decline in sexual interest and enjoyment as married heterosexual women. In fact, lesbians said this was prime time for them sexually. Given that, it is important to look at the differences between heterosexual and lesbian relationships. One of the things that may be different is the nature of power in the relationship—how you talk about things and who is in charge. If you are in a relationship with a man and experiencing decreased sexual interest, it may be time to look at it and negotiate ways to feel more excited about being in that relationship.

Although marriage offers the security of having a partner, it often breeds assumptions about partner responses, accompanied by specific expectations, especially if you have been married a long time. Women may feel afraid that they are becoming unattractive as they get older and let their emotions fester without even consulting their husbands for an updated opinion.

Whether married, single, heterosexual, or lesbian, if you are interested in enhanced sexual enjoyment, you need to take a perhaps scary, but powerful, step in introducing changes into relationships, talking with your partner, and feeling in charge.

Menopausal Sex Therapy

For those women not willing to let menopausal changes affect their sex lives, there are myriad options available. These are proven solutions that work for many women, and the majority of them are not drug related. Be open-minded and give them a try.

Reversing Vaginal Dryness

Successful treatment of vaginal dryness falls into three categories: hormone replacement therapy, lubricants, and regular sex.

Hormone Replacement Therapy. Vaginal dryness and hot flashes are the two complaints that bring most women to a doctor's office requesting hormone replacement therapy. Although there are pluses and minuses involved (see Chapter 4, "Hormone Replacement Therapy"), hormone replacement therapy is very effective in treating vaginal dryness. Successfully prescribed, hormone replacement therapy

- Restores lubrication to the vagina.
- Thickens the vaginal lining, making it less prone to irritation.
- Reduces the incidence of vaginal and urinary tract infections.

Dr. Lila Nachtigall, associate professor of obstetrics and gynecology at New York University Medical Center and a pioneer in hormone replacement therapy research, believes successful hormone replacement therapy treatment is achieved when a woman has comfortable sex and no more than one or two vaginal or urinary tract infections a year. An advocate of the appropriate use of hormone replacement therapy, Dr. Nachtigall strongly recommends it for patients with uncomfortable vaginal changes if no medical reason contraindicates its use. She says, "Estrogen has saved untold marriages and relationships and made others possible."

Lubricants. Look no farther—Mother Nature has provided the best lubricant of all: saliva. Nothing fancy, either your own saliva or that of your partner is the easiest and most effective way to provide lubrication prior to intercourse. If oral sex does not appeal to your partner, saliva can easily be applied with the fingertips.

Beyond this option, many kinds of vaginal lubricants are available, and several manufacturers have made efforts to update and develop new products that closely imitate your own natural lubricant (see Chapter 2, "What's Going to Happen to Me? . . . Perimenopause"). All of this sounds good, but many women are uncomfortable with this solution: Either they have never used a lubricant, dislike touching their genitals, feel a sense of failure about their dryness, or are embarrassed to discuss the situation with their partner. This is a common problem but one that can be solved.

How do you introduce a lubricant into your sexual script with your partner? Do you just pass the tube of lubricant and say, "Here, honey, use some of this?" Not much of a turn-on.

A better strategy is to get familiar with lubricants yourself before you involve your partner. This will also give you a chance to explore pleasurable sexual techniques by performing self-stimulation. Based on the statistics, masturbation should not be a novel experience. It is practiced by the majority of women, continuing right into old age, with more than 25 percent of women in their 70s acknowledging this behavior.

Dr. Jamie Ostroff, a sex therapist and psychologist at Memorial Sloan-Kettering Cancer Center, suggests the following procedure for familiarizing yourself with lubricants and masturbation:

- Select one or more lubricants from your local pharmacy for testing. There are definite differences in the products, and buying several to try is a small investment in your sexual satisfaction.
- Choose a private and comfortable time when you are certain you will not be interrupted. Some women find it helpful to put on some music or a videotape with romantic or erotic scenes.
- Touch, smell, and taste the lubricant to select one you like and can feel comfortable using.

- Take a hot bath, relax, and set the stage to enjoy yourself.
- While in the bath, fantasize about a past pleasurable sexual encounter or one you would like to have. Imagine having sex with your partner or someone else you find attractive—this is a great time to have an imaginary affair. Think about whatever you find sexy and drop your inhibitions.
- After you get out of the bath and towel off, get a hand-held mirror and look at your genitalia. Many women have never looked closely at their genitals and are not familiar with their sexual organs and responses. Seeing firsthand is often helpful. However, if this makes you uncomfortable, skip it and go on to the next step.
- Squeeze out a dab of lubricant and touch it to the lips of your vagina as if you were moisturizing it. Pay attention to the sensations this produces. Add more lubricant to the lips and then to the inside of the vagina; add a lot of lubricant onto your clitoris and the surrounding area. Continue to stimulate and massage the area, experimenting with different rhythms and pressures. Women who have not been able to achieve orgasm, even for many years, find that just one to three minutes of stimulation around the hood of the clitoris can result in orgasm.

After you have experimented with a lubricant, give some thought as to how you might tell your partner about it as well as any personal discoveries you have made about your sexual response. Ideally, lubricants should be part of foreplay. For heterosexual couples, place some lubricant on your partner's penis and stroke it; most men will love this. In fact, a lot of men will probably be more open to using a lubricant than most women. After all, any extra attention devoted to your partner will undoubtedly be appreciated.

Regular Sex. Sexual intercourse at least once a week is still the most effective drug-free way to relieve vaginal dryness. However, it is not uncommon to find yourself in a situation where regular sex just is not possible—no partner, poor health, no desire. Fortunately, there are several ways to remedy this condition and maintain a healthy, well-lubricated vagina.

Kegel exercises, which are also useful to prevent urinary stress incontinence, are particularly helpful, especially when combined with a habit of self-stimulation. Ideally, Kegel exercises should be performed by all women throughout their lives to ensure a physically fit urogenital area. You are probably asking, What next? However, Kegels are easy to do and undetectable when you are doing them. Simply tighten your muscles as if to stop the flow of urine and then release. It is best to tie these exercises to a daily activity, such as completing ten Kegels every time you brush your teeth. For more detailed instruction, see the section on urinary stress incontinence in Chapter 2, "What's Going to Happen to Me? . . . Perimenopause."

Another way to deal with the absence of a partner and maintain your sexual response is to use a device called a vaginal dilator or penis replica. This is not a dildo or vibrator, although it has the same shape. Vaginal dilators come in different sizes to accommodate the various sizes of women's vaginas and can be purchased at a pharmacy or surgical supply store. They also come in a variety of colors. The technique is simple: Apply lubricant to the dilator, insert it into your vagina, and do a couple of repetitions of Kegel exercise sets. This will give your muscles a real workout.

Despite the fact that vaginal dilators are most often recommended for women who have had radiation treatment to their pelvis, cervix, or vagina, they provide benefits for women who have not undergone this procedure. If you go for many months without a sexual relationship in your life, it becomes very important to avail yourself of a dilator, even temporarily. By using the dilator three times a week, you will be able to prevent vaginal shrinkage. Dilators work best when used early; do not wait until your vagina becomes totally dry and tight.

Although you can derive sexual pleasure from a dilator, using one is not necessarily the same thing as masturbating. Even if you dislike masturbation, you can use a dilator without creating strong sexual sensations, much the same way as you use a tampon. Try to feel comfortable about making dilation a lifelong habit.

No More Painful Sex

Simply put, every episode of painful sex decreases desire in women and can lead to what sex therapists call "spectatoring." This happens when a woman is not wholeheartedly involved in the sexual encounter and almost watches herself perform. In cases of *dyspareunia*, or painful sex, a woman is watching anxiously for any hints of pain and waiting for intercourse to be over. Pleasure is not even on the priority list. Unfortunately, this kind of behavior can turn into a vicious cycle—apprehension makes your muscles tense up, which can make intercourse painful. You expect it to be painful, so it is.

The best way to compensate for dyspareunia is to spend a sufficient amount of time in foreplay and to allow for appropriate arousal and vaginal lubrication. Use a vaginal lubricant if you need to. Most importantly, let your partner know about your need to lengthen foreplay activity.

In some instances after a period of painful sex, sex therapists advise their patients to avoid intercourse for a while, although they do not prohibit orgasm achieved through other sexual activity. This technique can ease a woman back into sexual relations and help her overcome her fears as well as those of her partner about hurting her. During this limited time of no intercourse, there are a host of other activities to focus on for sexual fulfillment: mutual masturbation, oral sex, or just holding each other and being intimate. In addition to improving circulation and enhancing relaxation, touching each other for extended periods of time can be highly erotic. This is a great opportunity to play with feathers, fur, scented oils, or other delectable treats. Try this regimen for a week or so, avoiding penetration until around the ninth day. By that time you should feel relaxed, confident, and enthusiastic about intercourse.

The worst thing for women experiencing vaginal dryness is quickie sex: "We're late for dinner." Or "The movie starts in an hour. Let's have a quickie." What worked well when you were younger and lubricated quickly may not fit your situation at midlife. In fact, quickie sex in these circumstances can often lead to disappointment and possibly pain.

A final note: Women should not have painful sex. Not being honest and coming clean with your partner about what hurts is worse than faking an orgasm. You do not want to be in a position of covering up and admitting later, "It's hurt all these years and I've never told you." You have a variety of options—try them.

Relief for Low Libido

Although the focus of menopausal changes often centers around the decline of estrogen, another hormone in your body is also affected, namely, testosterone. Produced by the ovaries and adrenal glands, testosterone, known as a female androgen, has been shown to affect libido.

A British study published in 1977 found that estrogen plus testosterone significantly improved libido in 80 percent of women who complained of loss of libido after hysterectomy. Likewise, in a study of women who had surgical menopause with removal of both ovaries, conducted by Dr. Barbara Sherwin of McGill University, a combination of estrogen and testosterone boosted sex drive, arousal, and sexual fantasizing, whereas placebo and estrogen alone did not. The women who took estrogen and testosterone were comparable to a group of women who underwent hysterectomy without removal of their ovaries.

Based on the results of this study, Dr. Winnifred Cutler, author of *Hysterectomy: Before and After* (New York: Harper & Row, 1988) and founder of the Athena Institute for Women's Wellness, concludes, "The effectiveness of testosterone replacement therapy in restoring sexual interest after ovariectomy shows that androgens may stimulate sexual interest in women in much the same way they do in men."

Consequently, some doctors now assess a woman's testosterone level if she reports reduced sex drive, regardless of whether or not she still has her ovaries. Not a precise indicator, normal levels of testosterone range between 30 and 90 nanograms per milliliter, an enormous spread. If you have a testosterone reading of 90 nanograms per milliliter before menopause and it drops to 30 nanograms per milliliter after, however, you will most likely notice a decrease in your sex drive. Clinically, doctors define female androgen deficiency as a level less than 30 nanograms per milliliter.

If your tests indicate low levels of testosterone, you may want to investigate some of the new preparations of estrogen replacement that also include low doses of testosterone. An added benefit of this therapy is the relief of breast tenderness experienced by some women on estrogen.

As you might expect, there are some troublesome side effects to taking testosterone, even in small doses: facial and chest hair growth, acne, deepening of the voice, and perhaps liver damage. Most critically, testosterone can increase cholesterol levels and raise your risk for cardiovascular disease.

Still in its infancy, testosterone replacement research is centered on finding answers to critical issues. Suitable doses and types of testosterone are unknown. The exact effects on sexuality are unclear, and doctors do not know just what testosterone does to a woman's body.

This means that even if you decided to try testosterone replacement, you will probably be faced with months of dosage adjustments and side effects. It may be worth the effort to give it a try, but understand that you will have to stay on top of your treatment and do as much research as you can on the subject. The bottom line: Testosterone replacement to treat libido is a controversial therapy.

Communication: The Key to Good Sex

With all of the changes happening to your body and perhaps your partner's as well, you would have to be a fairly flexible and communicative person to keep up. Sexual dysfunction, both male and female, is quite common at 50. Unless you make the effort to understand and cope with the changes, your sex life may get left in the dust.

> *There's a part of me that asks myself, "Are we not having sex more often because my husband has some feelings about menopause?" And I'm not asking him. It's funny because in a lot of ways I feel more sexual than I have for a long time. But I can see that this is something I need to talk to him about.*
>
> Married mother, 50

Start with your sexual routine. You know, the one that has worked for you for years. Chances are it could use a little re-working once you reach midlife. Longer periods of foreplay are necessary to achieve sexual arousal. A shift away from intercourse toward other forms of intimacy is important. Many women are not as interested in intercourse as men, perhaps because only 50 percent achieve orgasm regularly with intercourse. Older men can experience erectile difficulties and are not as wedded to ejaculation as they were when they were younger. Take a close look at your routine and see how it fits your changing needs and interest. More importantly, get some input from your partner so that you are not left in the dark about what is really going on.

> *I often wonder about my husband's libido. If I'm unable or not in the mood to have intercourse for an extended period of time, he doesn't complain. It's not that we give up having sex, it's just that sometimes we tailor it down quite a bit. How come he's able to give up having intercourse? He's four years older than me, and I suspect he's not as interested anymore. Otherwise I think he would be more enthusiastic about creative lovemaking, especially when I'm incapacitated. If his sex drive was the same as when he was younger, he'd be begging for more.*
>
> Married mother, 52

If you are not doing so on a regular basis, now is the time to establish good communication with your mate. According to

Deborah Edelman, author of *Sex in the Golden Years* (New York: Donald I. Fine, 1992), "It has been documented that simply discussing sex can do more to alleviate sexual problems—from inhibition to impotence—than considerably more ambitious psychotherapeutic, behavioral, and other educational methods." Talking relieves anxiety and misconceptions. However, it is far easier to have a discussion if you know what you are talking about, so start your sexual odyssey after menopause by reading about sexual techniques and response. Encourage your partner to do the same (see Appendix 2, "Resources").

This woman and her husband are in desperate need of renewed communication and an updated sexual scenario.

I think we're missing out on a good sex life, I really do. It's awful hard to go through lovemaking without really making love, if you know what I mean. You can't put fifteen minutes or half an hour away to just smooch or something like that. If I'm out of commission for one reason or another, my husband is usually left out in the cold. He's definitely old-fashioned and inhibited, gets embarrassed easily, and doesn't like oral sex. He's not the type to just lie there and say, "Do me."

Married woman, 45

Despite the sexual revolution of the past twenty to thirty years, people may be talking more but not communicating about the issues that are truly important. Even in couples who claim to have a good sex life, there is very little real communication about personal sexual preferences. As simple as it sounds, talking to your partner or your doctor about sex can be almost impossible for many women. Years of conditioning that sex talk is taboo or just an embarrassment can rob you of your power of speech. Unless you feel you have a sensitive, receptive, nonjudgmental audience, you may have trouble saying a single word, just like this woman married for over twenty-five years.

We don't have sex as often and I can tell my husband's not happy about it. I always find excuses—a headache, a stomachache—I guess I'm not being honest about my lack of interest. But what else can I do? You can't have a huge discussion every time my husband wants sex. So I guess it will have to be excuses, but he's been very patient. Not being open and talking about it is probably the coward's way out. I know talking to him would really be the right thing to do.

Married mother, 55

Here are some guidelines to get your verbal juices flowing. Psychologist Dr. Mardell Grothe, who works extensively with couples to improve communication in relationships, often uses the following problem-solving techniques in his practice. Dr. Grothe says, "While many of these suggestions may seem counterintuitive, they work. The key is to be patient, caring, open, and un-self-centered in working through your problems."

- *The first step is to enlist your partner in a problem-solving effort.* You both need to come to some sort of agreement that you want to achieve a greater sense of harmony, satisfaction, and intimacy with each other. If you do not make this agreement, nothing you attempt subsequently will work.
- *Next, learn more about your partner's sexual needs and preferences.* "What about me?" you may ask. "I'm feeling hurt, wounded, and slighted, and sometimes my partner doesn't even care about my needs. And you're asking me to figure out what my partner wants?" The answer is yes. This is not the time for a self-centered attitude, no matter how badly you feel.

  Right now, it is critical to ferret out what is important to your partner. You will probably get some useful information and certainly a different viewpoint from your own. Unless you air issues that may be preoccupying your partner, it will be difficult for your partner to be sensitive to your problems. Given this kind of attention, your partner will then be far more receptive to hearing and meeting your needs. Think of this as the relationship equivalent of "Ask not what your country can do for you . . ."

- *Put theory into practice.* Understanding this viewpoint is easy, but doing it can be very difficult. Someone has to make the first step, and since you are the one reading this book, why not try? You cannot just go to your partner and say, "Look, I've got some needs that you're not meeting—I'm not blaming you for this, by the way—and we need to talk about them so I'll be happier." It just does not work that way. You are not the only person in this relationship who may have issues with your sex life.

  Instead, try a more evenhanded approach, something like, "I want to have a sex life with you where we both feel like we're getting what we want. And I'm not so sure I know exactly what you want and need from me. There are also times when I don't think you know what I want either. I just want to sit down and talk about it and see what I can do to make you happier."

- *Create an atmosphere in which your partner feels safe to talk.* This is not the time to play "the blame game," although that certainly seems like the easiest way to handle things. Restrain yourself and set up a nonconfrontational environment where you can talk without being interrupted.

- *View this as a process, not an event.* Try not to approach this kind of communication as a one-shot deal. There is too much at stake if you set it up as a single event and it does not work out. This is a process that can occur over time. You can stop it when you want and pick it up again when it seems appropriate. If you start talking and it looks like you or your partner are not in a flexible or understanding mood, it might be a good idea to cut the conversation short and resume it later in the week.

  Do not expect total agreement. This is an iterative process that will involve a lot of give and take. One of the benefits of multiple conversations is that it gives you both time to think. Your partner may flat out disagree with what you say today. However, it is not uncommon to have a complete change of heart once your partner has had time to think about it for a while. Be reasonable in your expectations and do not expect results overnight.

- *Talk less and communicate more.* No matter how hard they try, some people just do not want to talk about sex. It inhibits them and makes them feel uncomfortable. The goal of this process is not talking about sex. It is about you and your partner feeling more satisfied that you are meeting each other's needs in an intimate context.

The difference between when we were first married and now is that we are able to talk to each other in a different way. We are not as protective of our feelings. We're also more sexually intimate than we used to be, which gives us both a lot more freedom.

Married mother, 52

Some couples exchange books on various subjects in an effort to express their views and then never talk about them. Instead, they may adopt some of the ideas and techniques from their reading and weave them into their lovemaking. Partners, in turn, respond with positive feedback to encourage repeat behavior, and not a single word may be spoken.

If you have the courage to speak out, make sure your thoughts are clear and well organized. This does not mean rehearsing for hours in front of a mirror. The last thing you need in talking with your partner is an inflexible script. More likely than not, it was just this kind of inflexibility that set up a barrier between this woman and her husband when she tried to have a discussion.

I've talked to my husband about menopause and vaginal dryness and my waning interest in sex, but he's not a particularly introspective person. I gave one or two speeches where my sole intent was to let him know that none of this was his fault and that he's just as attractive to me as ever. I think he understands, but I know he's disappointed. Every once in a while he alludes to the fact that sex was fun while it lasted.

Married mother, 50

If you are a good listener, you may want to change some of your original thinking once you have heard what your partner has to say. Be open and caring. Your thoughts should come from your heart, not your head.

Sex After Hysterectomy and Cancer Therapy

You're not supposed to be stuck like this—stuck with someone who's not really a woman.
—thirtysomething character Nancy Weston to
her husband after hysterectomy and
ovariectomy for ovarian cancer

Physical and Emotional Factors

Women who enter premature or abrupt menopause as a result of hysterectomy or cancer surgery have more and severe sexual problems than any other group of women. According to recent research, sexual difficulties are almost inevitable after these procedures and women report declines in sexual frequency, satisfaction, and capability.

The level of impact on your sex life is usually predicated by the type of procedure involved. Removal of your ovaries during hysterectomy or total ovarian shutdown as a result of chemotherapy can have a devastating effect. Suddenly and abruptly, vital hormone production stops. Even if you retain your ovaries after hysterectomy, evidence suggests that removal of the uterus may contribute to vaginal dryness, scarring, and decreased genital sensation.

The effect of these medical interventions on your sex life goes beyond the physical. Emotional issues associated with hysterectomy and cancer therapy raise huge questions about sexuality and identity:

- How you feel about yourself, whether or not you are depressed.
- How comfortable you are with yourself and the changes in your body.
- How easily you can relax and feel sexual again.
- How much energy you have if you are undergoing energy-zapping treatments like chemotherapy.
- What side effects you may be experiencing, like masculinizing effects of some hormone treatments.
- The fear sex will hurt.
- Anxiety over whether you will still be attractive to your partner.
- Whether you will be able to attract a partner at all.

Studies have shown that sexual difficulties after hysterectomy or cancer treatment may be due to preexisting depression or to the fear that this kind of surgery will result in a loss of attractiveness and diminished sexual satisfaction.

Getting Back on Track
You can still have a pleasurable, sensual, sexual experience after surgery and treatment, particularly if you are motivated and have a reasonably supportive partner. Surgery can present an opportunity to talk with a partner about sex for the first time. Even though you may feel done in or not in control as a result of your surgery, it can empower you to relearn sexual pleasure—just like when you were a teenager.

Regaining your sex life comes down to a combination of courage and communication. Spontaneous sex may not be possible right away. If you think about it, though, the cast-all-caution-to-the-wind philosophy of early sexual encounters was probably replaced long ago by more prearranged sexual activity. The most important point is to get started. It is much better to get your sex drive up and running as soon after surgery as you are able. The longer you wait, the more chance you have of developing problems and inhibitions.

Although resuming sexual activity is important, sufficient time for healing is needed. Because the body is bruised from surgery, it may take several months before you can enjoy sex again and not just tolerate intercourse. However, 50 percent of women who undergo hysterectomy and are in a stable heterosexual relationship are sexually active within two months; 90 percent resume their sex lives within four months.

Your first attempts at renewed lovemaking may be disappointing. Do not get discouraged. In a way, this is unchartered territory. You may need to remind your partner to be especially gentle at first, particularly when stimulating the genital area. Extreme genital sensitivity will disappear after a few weeks of gentle stimulation.

The American Cancer Society recommends the following approach to prevent pain during sexual activity after cancer procedures or hysterectomy:

- Plan sexual activity for the time of day when your pain is weakest.
- Find a position for touching or intercourse that puts as little pressure as possible on the painful areas of your body.
- Focus on your feelings of pleasure and excitement and not on pain.

With all these changes happening to your body, you may also experience orgasm in a different way. You may even have to relearn how to actually have an orgasm and develop new techniques for achieving one. Unaccustomed feelings during sexual contact are common and will probably require some adjustment. Even with all of these unfamiliar sensations, however, you should still be able to have an orgasm.

Your partner will also need a great deal of reassurance and new information. Men, in particular, will be afraid of hurting you and harbor the illusion, as most men do, that they are responsible for your pleasure. Help out your partner by offering relevant information on menopause and the effects it is having on your body. Avoid this kind of conversation after a bout of unsuccessful lovemaking. Instead, take it up at a less emotionally charged time and be sure to discuss any sexual difficulties your partner may also be experiencing.

For women who have surgically or chemically induced menopause, one of the most common complaints, as with other menopausal women, is the loss of sexual desire. Although you may not experience it right away, almost half of all women who undergo hysterectomy, regardless of whether or not their ovaries are removed, report a loss of libido. This may be a result of emotional issues or due to drastically lowered testosterone levels. As discussed earlier, you may want to ask your doctor to check your testosterone level and see if you could benefit from testosterone replacement. Most of the studies of testosterone replacement involved women who had their ovaries removed. Contrary to popular belief, estrogen replacement alone will not increase your sexual desire. However, the majority of women on appropriate hormone replacement do report a normal degree of sexual desire and function after hysterectomy.

Chemotherapy and Your Sex Life
Going through surgery and chemotherapy for cancer is an ordeal and the last thing you want to hear is that you will experience premature menopause on top of everything else. Unfortunately, this is the case for most women. Some of them will be able to find some relief by taking hormone replacement therapy, although higher dosages are usually needed to be effective. Other women might also need testosterone replacement. Some women may be prohibited from taking any replacement hormones due to their condition. All of this can make a difficult situation even harder.

Take the loss of libido, for example. Women on chemotherapy often lose their desire for sex because the side effects are so draining. They are usually nauseous and weak after treatments and may feel unattractive due to weight and hair loss. Fortunately, sexual desire typically returns after chemotherapy, as the side effects slowly fade.

I truly don't know if my sex drive is any different after all this chemotherapy and radiation. I think I am far more likely to fall asleep when I hit the bed than I was before all this started. Is that a function of estrogen level or is it a function of what has been done to my body? I'm 48 years old . . . 48-year-old people don't stay up around the clock.

Married woman, 48

For women with cancer, there is also the persistent psychic trauma that your body has failed you. The sudden cessation of menstruation is a poignant reminder. All of this can affect sexuality and have a devastating effect on younger women. This is an area of treatment that needs some serious research.

Pregnancy and Contraception

"It ain't over till it's over" should be the motto of women approaching menopause. During perimenopause, you may notice irregular periods, think that you are home free, and dispense with all forms of contraception. This is definitely a premature strategy. Irregular periods are not an indication of loss of fertility and many women continue to ovulate during this time. This means you are still at risk of becoming pregnant, yet surveys indicate that approximately one in five women over 40 use no method of birth control.

Some Sobering Statistics
To gain perspective on the seriousness of the issue of birth control, especially for women over 40, take a look at the following:

- Each year, more than 50 percent of pregnancies in the United States are unintended, the highest rate in the developed world.
- These 3.5 million unintended pregnancies result in approximately 1.5 million unintended births, 1.6 million legal abortions, and 440,000 miscarriages.

- The United States has one of the Western world's highest abortion rates at 325 abortions per 1,000 live births.
- The incidence of elective abortions of pregnancies in women over 40 is among the highest of all age groups.

The ramifications of a cavalier attitude toward contraception in your 40s are obvious. Unless deliberately trying to conceive, most women who become pregnant in their 40s are not happy with the situation.

Contraception Options

It is clear that if you continue to be sexually active in the perimenopausal years, you must also continue to utilize contraception. Fortunately, all the options you had before—withstanding any personal contraindications—are still available to women in their 40s and 50s.

Birth Control Pills. In a recent ruling, the FDA revised its position and deemed low-dose birth control pills safe for women in their 40s *if* you are healthy, do not have any contraindications to the Pill, and are a nonsmoker. The FDA feels strongly that the benefits of the Pill outweigh the risks and that for women in their 40s the Pill is safer than pregnancy.

It is not surprising that many doctors now advocate the FDA's decision and enthusiastically prescribe oral contraceptives. Now commonly referred to as "the transition pill," it is used by women until they reach their late 40s, at which time they are switched over to hormone replacement therapy. This strategy can make perimenopause and menopause a breeze for certain women. With this therapy they will avoid pregnancy and hot flashes and, at the same time, help maintain bone density. Irregular menstrual bleeding, one of the top reasons for D&Cs and hysterectomies in women over 40, can also be avoided.

There are more benefits beyond the relief of the signs of menopause. Birth control pills protect against endometrial and ovarian cancer, pelvic inflammatory disease, anemia, rheumatoid arthritis, benign breast disease, and functional ovarian cysts.

Pill use has also been associated with the relief of PMS, which is frequently more severe after age 35.

The downside is that there is still uncertainty about the link between breast cancer and the Pill, despite rigorous research. Nevertheless, most doctors feel the risk of breast cancer with Pill use is negligible and is offset by the reduction in ovarian and endometrial cancer.

For women who cannot tolerate estrogen, three progestin-only options are available. There are progestin-only pills; Norplant, a five-year contraceptive that is implanted in your upper arm; and Depo-Provera injections, which last three months. These methods protect women against endometrial cancer and are quite effective in preventing pregnancy. (Although Depo-Provera is used as a contraceptive in more than ninety countries worldwide, it has not been approved by the FDA for birth control because of a possible link to breast cancer. Nevertheless, it is still prescribed by some doctors in the United States.) All three progestin-only methods can stop menstruation or cause irregular menstrual bleeding and may cause significant depression in sensitive women.

Intrauterine Devices (IUDs). Underutilized in the United States, IUDs are an ideal form of birth control for many women in mutually monogamous relationships. Unfortunately, many women still remember the problems associated with the Dalkon Shield, which has been off the market for years, and view the IUD as a dangerous prospect. Today, there are two IUDs available in the United States: the Copper T380A, which provides eight years of birth control, and the newer Progestasert, which provides one year. Failure rates are low, and complications are minimal but can include pain with intercourse and vaginal bleeding. Women who do use IUDs rate them highly.

Sterilization. The number one contraceptive choice of couples over the age of 35 is still sterilization. For women this usually means a tying off of the fallopian tubes, called *tubal ligation*, which prevents an egg from being fertilized. Referred to as a simple procedure, it can often have complications that may result in heavy monthly bleeding, irregular cycles, and long periods of flow. Trauma to your pelvic area created by this procedure can also affect the function of your ovaries by decreasing hormonal production and making ovulation irregular. Given these realities, it is important to investigate the various procedures used in tubal ligation and gain a thorough understanding of the pluses and minuses.

For men, sterilization in the form of a vasectomy is a less risky proposition with few, if any, repercussions. Perhaps because of a misplaced macho mentality, many men erroneously think a vasectomy will affect their sexual performance or detract from their masculine image. This is not a form of castration. A vasectomy is a simple twenty-minute procedure, done under local anesthetic. It is performed on thousands of men every year with great success.

Dr. Penny Wise Budoff, in her ground-breaking book on menopause, *No More Hot Flashes,* discusses sterilization in great detail and recommends tubal ligation only in the following circumstances:

- Your partner refuses to have a vasectomy.
- Using the Pill or an IUD is too risky because of current health status or history.
- You have had failures with barrier methods (condom, spermicide, or diaphragm) or have an aversion to their use.
- The prospect of pregnancy is disastrous for you.
- Your general health is good.

Take your time with this decision. Sterilization is usually irreversible.

Staying Sexy and Safe

For menopausal women without partners, sex with another person can be a difficult prospect. Some women find themselves suddenly single for a variety of reasons and quake at the thought of dating again after a hiatus of many years. Other women, familiar with being single, may balk at dealing with sexual relationships and the effects of menopause. In either case, the techniques mentioned in this chapter— self-stimulation, hormone replacement therapy, Kegel exercises, and the use of lubricants and vaginal dilators—will go a long way to ensure good sexual health.

How do you actually approach a new relationship when you are menopausal? The answer is: very carefully, honestly, and patiently. According to sex therapist Dr. Derek Polonsky, "Having a new love later in life can be every bit as anxiety producing as it was in the late teens or early 20s. The same concerns about being accepted and feeling competent arise. Only time and trust ease those worries." So be reasonable about your expectations and take things slowly. Your prospective partner is probably suffering some of the same fears and uncertainty.

Faced with dating and menopause, this single mother was afraid to initiate communication.

I've been dating this man for a while and have avoided talking about menopause and my lack of sexual desire. He seems to be accepting me for what I am without making any value judgments. But at some level he has to be aware of what's happening. I mean, he's seen my menopause books lying around and we've talked about the fact that I don't have much energy, sexual or otherwise. I guess I feel a little ashamed to talk about menopause in detail. And I have a feeling that if I talk about it too much, he'll get frustrated and bored and leave me.

Single mother, 49

Although this is an understandable dilemma, the next step is to take some risks and begin a dialogue. Approaching your partner about what is important to him will probably get you off to a good start. For more details on the significance of menopause from a male viewpoint, see Chapter 9, "Men and Menopause."

In addition to overcoming any sexual inhibitions, you now

need to be concerned about sexually transmitted diseases (STDs) and AIDS. STDs are not just for kids, and AIDS is quickly spreading into the heterosexual and lesbian population. When you make love with a new partner, you are each having sex with all of your previous partners. It only takes one act of unprotected intercourse to transmit STDs and AIDS. And men are far more likely to transmit venereal diseases to women than vice versa.

Statistics on AIDS are always frightening, but the increase in the number of women being affected is startling. According to the Centers for Disease Control, AIDS cases among women living in the United States have increased by 37 percent in the past year, with 24,323 American women with AIDS. Worse still, the projected number of HIV (human immunodeficiency virus) infections among women worldwide by the year 2000 is 15 to 20 million.

Make the following safe sex tips part of your life and think of them as mandatory as opposed to helpful suggestions. No burning passion is worth the risk of STDs or AIDS.

- Use condoms, along with a contraceptive product containing the spermicide nonoxynol 9, which kills many STDs. Some condoms are lubricated with nonoxynol 9; otherwise use spermicidal foam, jelly, or suppositories in tandem with condoms. The Pill, progestin-only methods, IUDs, and withdrawal do not protect against most STDs and AIDS. Short of abstinence, condoms, spermicides, diaphragms, and sponges are the most effective guards against STDs.
- Do not engage in sexual relations with someone who has open sores on the genitals. Restrain yourself and wait until the sores are healed.
- If you think you are at risk, have an AIDS screening test. Many smart single adults will only have sex with partners who have been tested.
- Talk about STDs, past and present, with new partners.
- Discuss safe sex and monogamy. If you or your partner are not going to be monogamous, condoms and spermicide should be used indefinitely.

A Final Note

As you can see from the size of this chapter and the voices of
women featured throughout, sex is not a small issue for midlife
women. For more information check Appendix 2, "Resources."
Sex and intimacy after menopause can be an enriching part of
your life. Try not to let physical and emotional changes get in
the way.

Chapter Eight

Special Problems

Everything you have read so far focuses on the average woman and what she can expect during her menopausal years. However, some women just do not fall neatly into that category and have what are considered to be special problems. For them, menopause is often a completely different experience precipitated by an early, late, or even overnight cessation of monthly bleeding. Although these women usually experience familiar menopausal signs, they are often at greater risk for osteoporosis and heart disease, have more serious sexual problems and trouble with vaginal dryness, and suffer from severe emotional stress and trauma.

Specifically, women who have early spontaneous menopause, hysterectomy, chemically or radiation-induced menopause (usually related to cancer therapy), or late menopause have special problems and deserve special attention. So do women who have late pregnancies or a history of uterine fibroids.

Women in these situations are often at a distinct disadvantage. For example, because of the lack of user-friendly information, women with premature menopause are often caught unaware and unprepared. There is usually no one for them to talk to among their peers, and they end up feeling frightened and isolated. Women with surgically or chemically induced menopause have a similar dilemma. Their menopause is usually the by-product of treatment for a severe or life-threatening condition. Given the major trauma associated with these kinds of procedures, menopause and its own special set of potential problems are considered to be at the bottom of the list of considerations. When dealing with immediate and critical health concerns, long-term medical issues like osteoporosis and heart disease often fall by the wayside.

This chapter will provide you with a running start on being well informed about these special problems, help you to grapple with many complex issues, and aid in your decision making. Most importantly, it will establish the basis necessary for you to manage your special menopausal situation.

Early Menopause

This is a scary concept for the vast majority of women, but the term *early menopause* refers merely to menopause that occurs before the age of 51 in a nonconventional manner. A broad category, early menopause is usually associated with one of three precipitating events: spontaneous premature menopause, hysterectomy or surgically induced menopause, or chemically or radiation-induced menopause. Although the characteristics, statistics, and emotional implications of all three vary, the treatment options are similar and you will recognize many of the potential solutions.

Premature Menopause

Before women and doctors became even slightly knowledgeable about menopause, women experiencing normal perimenopause in their 40s were thought to be having "early menopause." Today, there is a greater understanding about the different phases of menopause and a 44-year-old woman with hot flashes might be considered to have an "earlier menopause."

This is not premature menopause. According to the experts, premature menopause is defined as happening to women under 40 years of age. It has all of the characteristics of regular menopause, including the end of your childbearing ability.

Unfortunately, this phenomenon is not as rare as you might think: Approximately 8 out of every 100 women experience premature menopause, also referred to as *premature ovarian failure*, before they turn 40. It can happen as early as the late teenage years, but usually occurs in women in their 20s or early 30s. These are women who have had regular periods and successful pregnancies all along. What a shock.

Imagine the feelings of this unsuspecting 39-year-old woman when she found out she was menopausal.

Becoming menopausal when I was 39 was one of the worse things that has ever happened to me. I wasn't prepared—who would be, and up until then I had been working with a fertility specialist trying to get pregnant. I'm feeling better now, not quite so emotional, but when it first happened I was a basket case. With the shock of menopause and the hormonal ups and downs that came with it, I wasn't fit to be with anyone. It's still difficult, and there are times when I think about it or talk with other people and I still cry. Not being able to have children is a loss in my life that I have to face every day. But I'm starting in vitro fertilization and have actively begun the adoption process. Early menopause is not going to keep me from being a mother.

Married woman, 41

Calculating the Odds

Not a total game of chance, premature menopause seems to be influenced by specific factors. It appears that women with a family history of premature menopause—a mother, grandmother, or sister who went through menopause before 40—are likely candidates. According to Dr. Charles Hammond, an obstetrician and gynecologist at Duke University Medical Center, "There does seem to be a tendency for age of mother and age of daughter at time of menopause to coincide. It's not a one-to-one direct relationship by any means, but there's a general agreement that if a mom's early, a daughter's early."

So use your family history as a guide. Even though she had the knowledge about her mother's menopause, this woman had difficulty accepting the evidence.

I can look back and see my mother going out onto our terrace in the dead of winter and throwing snow on her naked body because she was so hot. I was quite young and thought she was totally bizarre. She never told me it was related to menopause. As an adult, I remember my mother and older sister talking about hot flashes, comparing and contrasting their experiences. But it didn't dawn on me that I would follow in their footsteps. They both reached menopause in their very early 40s and so did I. I never quite understood that my mother had her symptoms so early, and when the same thing happened to my sister, I just ignored it. I assumed because we had such different lifestyles that menopause would not happen as early for me. Even though everyone in my family has followed the same pattern, it still came as a surprise.
Married woman, 42

Another influence on premature menopause is smoking, mentioned briefly in Chapter 1. Although opinions vary as to how many years a smoking habit will cut short your reproductive ability, doctors all agree that it will definitely have some effect. Some experts say smoking will cause menopause to occur two to three years earlier, and others say five to ten years. In his book *Managing Your Menopause* (New York: Prentice Hall, 1990), menopause authority Dr. Wulf H. Utian says two theories exist about smoking and earlier menopause: "One is that the contents of cigarette smoke cause the liver to destroy estrogen. The other suggests that nicotine reduces the blood supply to the ovary, which, lacking nourishment, may shrivel."

Rarely, immune disorders, such as lupus or Addison's disease, can cause women to produce antibodies that may affect the thyroid gland or ovarian tissue and result in premature menopause. Major invasive surgical procedures like hysterectomy and tubal ligation have also been thought to speed menopause by compromising blood circulation in the pelvic area.

Beyond the influence of these factors and chemotherapeutic drugs and radiation discussed later in this chapter, doctors do not have a clue as to the causes of premature menopause. This is not a comforting thought, but at least you now know the small amount of information that is out there and perhaps it will heighten your awareness and help with family planning decisions.

Menopausal Indicators

Premature spontaneous menopause is no different than menopause that occurs at the usual age of 51. Decreasing amounts of estrogen often precipitate fragmented sleep, hot flashes, night sweats, vaginal dryness, mood swings, and other annoying side effects. None of this happens overnight, and women with premature menopause can expect the same gradual progression of these menopausal indicators. Some women will experience them over a period of several years, and others may have them only for a short amount of time. However, according to records kept over a twenty-year period by the Reproductive Endocrine Unit of the Medical College of Georgia, women with premature menopause seem to experience milder menopausal symptoms as compared to older women.

To confirm your menopausal status, a measurement of your FSH level should be performed on day 1 of your cycle (see Chapter 1, "Are You Going Through Menopause?"). This is a blood test, taken each month for at least two consecutive months, and is considered to be more reliable than an estrogen measurement test in accurately determining your menopausal status. If your FSH level is raised appreciably, it is confirmation that your ovaries are no longer producing significant amounts of estrogen.

The Emotional Toll

Premature menopause can be a devastating diagnosis for a woman, especially if she has not yet realized a goal to be a mother. However, there are some extraordinary medical advances in the early development stages that may enable even a menopausal woman to become pregnant and carry a child to term. This is discussed briefly later in the chapter.

In addition to the childbearing issue, many women with premature menopause also experience embarrassment, anger, depression, and feelings of suddenly becoming an old lady. Some women say they feel singled out, much like a freak in a circus. Most women in this situation experience confusion about their sexuality and a loss of self-esteem.

The menopause newsletter *A Friend Indeed* did a special issue on premature menopause in February 1992 and reported: "The sense of loss is understandable but the irrational feelings of inadequacy which often accompany the loss are, for too many women, difficult to shed. We hear from young women who carry spare tampons for their friends, because they cannot bring themselves to admit that they no longer menstruate. We have letters from women plagued by feelings of inadequacy, but afraid to discuss it with a male partner for fear of driving him away. We have also heard from women who go from doctor to doctor looking for understanding and help."

However, some women, like this plucky 42-year-old who went through menopause in her late 30s, do not associate this major bodily change with a loss of femininity.

Early menopause hasn't really affected my identity as a woman, although I've come across a lot of other people in my situation who no longer feel like women. That just hasn't happened to me. I feel that I am who I am whether my hormones change or don't change or I bleed or I don't bleed or whether I have a child or I don't. I can even step back and enjoy not having my periods anymore—no cramps, no tampons, no mess.

Single woman, 42

Premature menopause is no picnic, and one of the most constructive things you can do is seek help and support. Menopause groups are springing up at hospitals and community centers and through various women's networks. Menopause clinics are also appearing throughout the country, often affiliated with large teaching hospitals in major cities. These clinics are often top-rate centers for information, exchange, and comfort. It can be well worth your effort to locate a clinic and try out some of its programs. Being informed, having the support of peers and professionals, and the passage of time can make all the difference in coping with premature menopause (see Chapter 10, "How to Get Good Treatment," and Appendix 2, "Resources").

Treatment with Hormone Replacement Therapy

Most doctors advocate hormone replacement therapy for women with premature menopause. For this group in particular, the evidence is strongest that hormone replacement therapy is very beneficial. According to Dr. Veronica Ravnikar, director of Reproductive Endocrinology, Fertility, Menopause at the University of Massachusetts Medical Center, "It's been clearly shown that women with premature menopause have a higher risk of heart disease and bone loss. So if any group is a clear candidate for hormone replacement therapy, this is the group—whether they went through menopause at a young age because their ovaries were removed or if they naturally went through an early menopause."

How long do you need to take estrogen? Many doctors believe that you should be on hormone replacement therapy until at least the age of biological menopause, 51. After that time, you are in the same situation as any other woman entering menopause at that age and can use the same criteria for making your decision (see Chapter 4, "Hormone Replacement Therapy").

Another approach is to examine your goals and expectations for hormone replacement therapy. If you focus on relieving hot flashes, a common estrogen-withdrawal phenomenon, it appears that two years is sufficient to get most women over the hump and into a hot-flash-free state. If your interest is in preventing osteoporosis, six years of hormone replacement therapy is usually recommended. However, when you stop, bone loss will occur, at which point it is advisable to have your bone density checked regularly (see Chapter 3, "Postmenopause"). Unfortunately, there is no clear recommendation for how long you should take hormone replacement therapy to lower your risk for heart disease.

In terms of dosage, although doctors prefer to start with the lowest dose of hormone replacement therapy possible, oftentimes prematurely menopausal women may need substantially more estrogen to relieve symptoms than do other women. Sometimes the dose of hormone replacement therapy actually needs to be doubled for prematurely menopausal women. "We start with the lowest dose possible," says Dr. Ravnikar, "but if after a period of time of about three to six months a woman is still having severe hot flashes, we can up the dose by double the amount."

There seems to be some question about whether doctors are undertreating young menopausal women. Doctors use the lowest bone-protective doses, but it is not clear if this is enough to protect against bone loss and heart disease in younger women and at the same time relieve vaginal dryness and other menopausal signs.

If a woman is very young, some doctors may suggest low-dose oral contraceptives rather than hormone replacement therapy. They serve the same purpose and may alleviate some of the emotional turmoil of a prematurely menopausal woman. Instead of taking a menopause drug, she can take a drug to prevent pregnancy, just like other women in the same age group.

Alternative Treatment
There are alternatives to hormone replacement therapy, but none of them has been studied long enough to provide a guarantee of their ability to protect against osteoporosis and heart disease, key issues for women experiencing premature menopause. However, there is no question that exercise and diet are critical factors. In fact, the American Heart Association has now declared lack of exercise to be a major risk factor for heart dis-

ease, ranking it equally with smoking, high cholesterol, and high blood pressure (see Chapter 5, "Alternative Treatment").

Surgically Induced Menopause (Hysterectomy)

Second only to cesarean section, hysterectomy—removal of the uterus—ranks as one of the most frequent forms of major surgery. One out of three women will have a hysterectomy, most likely in her 30s or 40s. These are staggering statistics and actually represent a 20 percent decline over the past couple of decades.

What is the story here? Why do so many women have hysterectomies? Do they all need them? Is almost every woman dysfunctional and unable to have a natural menopause?

Why Have a Hysterectomy?

According to the National Center for Health Statistics, approximately 600,000 hysterectomies are performed each year. In recent years, top reasons for hysterectomies have been fibroids, endometriosis, endometrial hyperplasia (excessive buildup of the uterine lining), cancer, and prolapse (falling down of the pelvic organs).

Typically, American doctors list as "appropriate reasons for hysterectomy" the following:

- Cancer of the pelvic organs.
- Severe, uncontrollable infection or bleeding.
- Life-threatening blockage of the bladder or intestines by the uterus or a growth in the uterus.
- A ruptured uterus.

Elective, but still appropriate, reasons include

- Precancers of the pelvic organs.
- Fibroids.

- Extensive endometriosis.
- Heavy uterine bleeding.
- Recurrent pelvic infections.
- Prolapse of the uterus.

Given these parameters, it is no surprise that more hysterectomies are performed in the United States than in Europe. It is also interesting to note that hysterectomy rates are much lower in the Northeast than in other sections of the country. *Consumer Reports* cites another rather disconcerting factor: "A woman is more likely to undergo a hysterectomy if her doctor is paid a fee for the surgery than if she belongs to a prepaid health plan."

Nevertheless, hysterectomy can be an obvious choice for many women who suffer from excessive bleeding over a long period of time and, in situations like the following, can make all the difference in the world.

I had been having a terrible time with my periods for the past year, and my doctor said I would have to have a hysterectomy sooner than later. But I resisted until one day, just before I was scheduled to go on vacation, I stood up and found myself standing in a pool of my own blood. It was the most frightening thing I've ever been through. In desperation and panic I called the doctor, who scheduled me for surgery that afternoon. I had just reached a point where I couldn't go on anymore. I couldn't wear anything light colored because I was always bleeding. I would walk around with a pocketbook full of overnight sanitary napkins or infant Pampers because I bled so heavily. I couldn't do anything strenuous. And I never went anywhere without being able to get in touch with someone to help me in an emergency. I really had no choice because I couldn't live that way one more day.

Married mother, 48

The tide seems to be turning against women just accepting hysterectomy as the solution for conditions like those mentioned above. They are starting to demand other alternatives like endometrial ablation—a process that uses a laser to destroy the uterine lining—to treat excessive bleeding, and myomectomy, a surgical technique for fibroid removal without loss of reproductive functioning.

Types of Hysterectomies

The term *hysterectomy* has evolved into a catchall phrase from its original context of removal of the uterus. Several types of hysterectomy exist today, and the terms can be confusing:

- *Total hysterectomy, also known as partial hysterectomy:* Removal of the uterus and cervix.
- *Total hysterectomy and bilateral salpingo-oophorectomy, also known as complete hysterectomy:* Removal of both ovaries, the fallopian tubes, uterus, and cervix. The term *salpingo* refers to the fallopian tubes; the word *oophorectomy*, to the ovaries. *Ovariectomy*, another term often used, is the same thing as an oophorectomy.
- *Subtotal (or subpartial or supracervical) hysterectomy:* Removal of the uterus only. It is rarely done today.

No matter what type of hysterectomy is prescribed, it is a major surgical procedure requiring general anesthesia. Surgery can be performed through an incision in the abdomen or through the vaginal opening. There are pluses and minuses with either approach, and you should make sure you have a clear understanding of them. There is also a good chance that you will be sick after a hysterectomy. In her book *Hysterectomy: Before and After*, Dr. Winnifred B. Cutler reports up to 70 percent of women undergoing hysterectomy experience postoperative illness. Common postoperative complications include infection; hemorrhage; and urinary, bowel, and vaginal problems. The aftereffects of hysterectomy can be very unpleasant.

The Ovary Issue

Given such a major medical procedure, it is amazing how little women know about the potential impact hysterectomy can have on their ovaries and, more importantly, the role ovaries play in a woman's immediate and long-term health picture. Believe it or not, many women undergoing hysterectomy neither ask nor know if their ovaries are being removed with their uterus. To give you some perspective, from 1985 to 1987, 45 percent of all women who had hysterectomies also had their ovaries removed; 55 percent did not. Broken down by age, a significant proportion of women under the age of 39 retained their ovaries after hysterectomy, 73 to 77 percent; after age 40, only 37 to 42 percent did.

The question of whether or not to have an oophorectomy is not a small detail to be overlooked or to be left automatically to the discretion of your doctor. The removal of your ovaries is a serious decision that should be made with all the information you can possibly get your hands on.

I had a hysterectomy and agreed to have my ovaries removed without really knowing what it meant. The best advice I can give to any woman contemplating a hysterectomy is to get a second and third opinion before you say, "Oh, yes, let's go ahead and take everything out." It never occurred to me how important my ovaries were and that if they were gone, I would have to do something radical to replace them . . . probably forever. Women should be really educated before they go to a doctor and agree to a hysterectomy. You may have to put up with bleeding a little longer or some other discomforts, but it may be worth it in the long run.
Married mother, 50

No matter how old you are, your ovaries can still be a vital part of your overall health outlook. Contrary to popular rumor, they do not shrivel up and become totally useless. Even after menopause, they may still produce small beneficial amounts of estrogen, and when that ends, they continue to produce testosterone. This means that your ovaries remain one of your first lines of defense against heart disease and osteoporosis. For example, in one study of 122,000 women who had undergone hysterectomy, the group of women who retained their ovaries had a significantly reduced risk of heart attack. Women who undergo hysterectomy and oophorectomy are seven times more likely to die of a heart attack than other women. In terms of the risk of osteoporosis, a woman of 50 without ovaries has the equivalent bone mass of a naturally menopausal woman of 70. Your ovaries also positively affect your arteries, skin, vagina, and sexual drive. Throw them out the window without a second thought? No, thank you.

Historically, doctors were taught that the ovaries became inactive after menopause and thus served no further purpose. Surgeons took that thinking one step further, assumed ovaries had no long-term value, viewed them as possible sites for disease, and routinely recommended removal during hysterectomy. However, because research has shown the ovaries' ability to continue to produce some hormones after menopause, many doctors have adopted a broader view on the issue.

Today, the decision about keeping your ovaries is often predicated on a woman's age, overall health, and family history. For women under 40 who are in good health, doctors usually recommend retaining the ovaries for the known benefits of protection against osteoporosis, lowering cardiovascular disease risk, and maintaining vaginal health and overall well-being. A woman in this situation—with ovaries and without a uterus—will no longer have monthly bleeding. Instead, eggs, if released from the ovaries, will simply be absorbed and dissolved by the body instead of making their way toward implantation in the womb.

Women in their 40s often fall into a gray area in the eyes of the medical community. Many doctors still feel that because these women have only a few years left until menopause, they might as well remove the ovaries. More enlightened doctors who understand the potential long-term benefit of retaining the ovaries take the opposite position. This can make decision making difficult. Your personal quest for more information from other sources may be extremely useful at this point.

I'm contemplating a hysterectomy and will probably have my ovaries removed, too. It's true that if you're under 40, they leave the ovaries in. If you're over 50, they take them out. In between, like me, they leave it to the patient to decide, which I feel is terribly unfair. They ask a layperson to make these decisions—how could I make the decision? My doctor said, "Get them out of there." Just his saying that, casually but emphatically, made the decision for me.

Married mother, 45

The biggest source of debate about ovary removal often centers around the issue of ovarian cancer. The image of Gilda Radner looms large in many women's minds and the prospect of eliminating this risk is often appealing. There is no question that ovarian cancer is a deadly, difficult to detect, and often incurable disease that claims 21,000 lives each year. However, the actual incidence of ovarian cancer is fairly low. According to Dr. William Hoskins, an ovarian cancer specialist at Memorial Sloan-Kettering Cancer Center, a woman's chance of getting ovarian cancer is only about 1.3 percent if there is no family history of the disease. Listed below are the risk factors for ovarian cancer:

- Strong family history of ovarian cancer—mother or sister.
- Previous incidence of colon, rectal, or breast cancer or a family history of such cancers or uterine cancer.
- Hereditary intestinal polyps.

Women with any of these factors are at a higher risk for ovarian cancer than other women and should probably opt for ovary removal during hysterectomy. Ideally, doctors should inform you of the pros and cons of ovary removal and encourage you to make your own decision. Doctors who advocate ovary removal to prevent ovarian cancer, especially if you do not fall into a high-risk group, are to be questioned closely.

As a general rule, Dr. Hoskins recommends the following for women with no ovarian cancer risk factors:

- *Under 40:* Keep your ovaries.
- *40 to 50 years old:* The decision is up to you.
- *Over 50:* Ovary removal is recommended.

If you are postmenopausal and decide to have your ovaries removed, it is unlikely that you will notice any immediate changes. Hormonal changes that occur as a result of ovary removal after menopause are subtle.

Although in most cases you should make every effort to retain your ovaries, if you have had breast cancer, you may want to readjust your thinking. Recent research suggests that oophorectomy after mastectomy slightly improves breast cancer survival in premenopausal women at ten years by 11 percent, whereas chemotherapy only improves it by 10 percent. Breast expert Dr. Susan Love, in *Dr. Susan Love's Breast Book* (New York: Addison Wesley, 1990), writes, "For premenopausal women with hormone-receptor-positive tumors and metastatic disease, oophorectomy has been the mainstay of treatment. Now we often use the estrogen blocker tamoxifen instead because of its limited side effects. They can also be used sequentially." Therefore, though controversial, some doctors may recommend knocking out the ovaries surgically or with radiation in breast cancer cases where prognosis is poor.

A final note on the issue of ovary removal. Most women, especially younger ones, receive hormone replacement therapy to compensate for loss of ovarian function after oophorectomy. Doctors feel that while replacement hormones are helpful, they are no substitute for the real thing. Dr. Lila Nachtigall and Joan Rattner Heilman confirm this in their book, *Estrogen* (New York: HarperCollins, 1991): "Most younger women without ovaries receive long-term estrogen replacement to make up for it, but one's own estrogen is always the best, not only because it is made by your own body, but because it is regulated according to your own individual day-to-day needs. ERT can never be as good as that."

After Hysterectomy

Recovery from hysterectomy can be slow and difficult. Routine as it may be to surgeons, it is still major surgery and a shock to your system. It can actually take up to a year for a woman to feel like she used to before surgery, which is longer than for most other operations.

Immediately after hysterectomy, even if you have retained one or both ovaries, it is not uncommon to experience hot flashes, night sweats, headaches, palpitations, depression, and dizzy spells due to a temporary interruption in blood flow and hormone production. Up to 70 percent of women undergoing hysterectomy have these problems. The symptoms typically occur suddenly on the second day after surgery and peak around the fourth or fifth day after surgery. As the recovery process continues and blood is restored, most of these symptoms disappear. Often doctors will prescribe estrogen to be taken during this time period while your body gets back to normal.

Another common side effect of hysterectomy is sexual discomfort, which occurs in 32 to 46 percent of cases, whether you have retained your ovaries or not. Sexual sensations and emotions change after hysterectomy, and it is important to be aware and ready to make some adjustments. You will undoubtedly feel battered and bruised inside after hysterectomy, and it may be three or four months before you can actually enjoy sexual intercourse. You may experience a temporary shrinking of your vagina or have pain from scar tissue as a result of the surgery. Even after tissues heal and tenderness abates, sexual problems may occur (see Chapter 7, "Sex").

There is also the possibility that one or both of your ovaries may fail after hysterectomy. This can occur within a few days after surgery or two to three years later. In theory, your ovaries should continue to function normally. However, interrupted blood supply to the organs or scar tissue may cause the ovaries to malfunction. In such cases, hysterectomy can lead to early menopause. Unfortunately, ovaries fail after one-third to one-half of all hysterectomies, either immediately or earlier than usual.

If you have had your ovaries removed, recovery from hysterectomy is somewhat similar but you have the additional problems associated with sudden menopause. No ovaries and no estrogen make for instant and absolute menopause. Because of the sudden drop in hormone levels, women without ovaries experience menopausal symptoms that are often more intense and long-lasting than after a natural menopause. All the usual symptoms occur a day or two after surgery, and the severity varies from woman to woman.

Whether or not the ovaries are retained after hysterectomy, removal of the uterus hastens the onset of menopause in 37 to 67 percent of women. This phenomenon seems to be related to age at the time of hysterectomy: The closer you are to natural menopause, the more likely the premature onset.

The Psychological Impact

Plainly speaking, hysterectomy, in all its varieties, is a form of castration. Although done for therapeutic reasons, it is still the removal of the reproductive organs. However, for some unknown reason, doctors rarely see it that way. When a man's testes are removed, it is called castration; when a woman's uterus, fallopian tubes, ovaries, or cervix are removed, doctors do not think of it as castration, but many women do.

> *I was trying to explain to my husband about why I felt so devastated about having a hysterectomy. I said, "How would you feel if you went in for an operation and afterward found out you had been left impotent?" Well, we were driving, and I thought he was going to crash the car. He said, "How could you say anything like that?" And I replied, "Because that's exactly how I feel."*
>
> Married mother, 48

Take Nancy Weston of television's *thirtysomething*, for example. Fed up with being treated like just another hysterectomized woman and feeling miserable, undesirable, and not a person anymore, Nancy railed at her gynecologist, "I've been castrated." Uncomfortable and indignant, he protested, telling her that was not the case at all. He insisted she had not been castrated and was obviously a little upset. Moreover, he told her she was entirely too aggressive about the whole thing. According to this doctor, Nancy would feel better once they had "played" with her estrogen dosage.

Society does not acknowledge the empty feeling of a woman who has had a hysterectomy. More so than women who go through premature menopause, hysterectomized women feel less than whole—their diseased organs needed to be cut out of their body. What is left is a big space where they used to have the potential to make a baby. Whether they wanted children or not, there is a sort of mourning for that loss.

Even in women who welcome the end of erratic periods or pain or the curing of cancer, surgically induced menopause often causes depression. A reminiscence by a 53-year-old woman printed in the March 1991 issue of *A Friend Indeed* shows how deeply affected one can be.

> When I arrived home, I opened a drawer and I caught sight of my last box of tampons. It felt like a stab in the heart; that part of me was now gone—not in the natural process I had anticipated, but in a single day of surgery. A crucial organ was absent and I would never be quite whole again. Isn't it significant that other amputations get such attention, while this hidden, gender-specific, but equally traumatic loss is virtually lost? At this low ebb, I heard of two friends, both happily pregnant, and felt a stab of envy . . . not jealousy, but strong nostalgia. I wanted to tell them to savor their time. I kept going, crying now and then, and gradually finished my mourning.

This same woman found a positive side to her hysterectomy plus oophorectomy, which was performed to remove a large fibroid. She lost weight, which was somewhat unusual, and she also found the certainty of menopause a benefit.

> I know exactly where I stand—no doubts about fertility, no question of hormonal status, my underwear is always presentable, my bedclothes unsullied. One must seek comfort in small things, right?

Though she tried to stay positive, she often found the tactless and insensitive remarks of other women a disappointment. It led her to think that there were not many who treasured womanhood; rather they looked upon it as an encumbrance or worse. Often meant to cheer, many remarks seemed flippant. It was evident that these women did not recognize gender as an important part of being a person. If surgical menopause was so sad for this nearly menopausal woman, it is often worse for younger women.

Depression is quite common, particularly in women who lose their ability to bear children before their time or before they have had a chance to conceive. This seems reasonable, but in fact, women who have no desire to be pregnant also suffer from depression after hysterectomy.

Research suggests that a significant percentage of hysterectomized women suffer a bout of severe depression within two or three years of the surgery. Hysterectomy seems to be associated with depression more than other types of surgeries.

According to Dr. Gloria Bachmann of the Robert Wood Johnson Medical School, counseling women about hysterectomy and the potential physical and psychological effects appears to help prepare them for the surgery and prevent postoperative problems. Still, women with a history of depression, sexual dysfunction, or other psychological disturbances have been shown in studies to have an increased prevalence of postoperative psychosexual problems after hysterectomy. Women who are uncertain about their desire for future pregnancies or who do not understand how the uterus functions or what the procedure entails are also at a greater risk for problems.

Based on a study of 8,000 Massachusetts women between 45 and 55 years old, it also appears that women who have had hysterectomies are subject to more chronic illnesses than are women who undergo natural menopause. Surgically menopausal women use twice as many prescribed drugs—sleeping pills, tranquilizers, and hormones—as naturally menopausal women and are more likely to consider their health worse than that of others. According to study author epidemiologist Sonja J. McKinlay, the stereotype of the "typical" menopausal woman is really drawn from her atypical sister—a woman whose menopause was caused by a surgeon, not biology.

Determining the Onset of Menopause

Without a uterus, you will no longer have a monthly menstrual period. This means you will also have to look for indicators other than cessation of menses to determine when you become menopausal. Women who have had hysterectomies and maintained one or both of their ovaries will experience the same kind of menopausal indicators as other women. It may happen slightly earlier than the average age of 51—although that is disputed by some doctors—but the signs will be the same. You may have hot flashes, sleep disturbances, vaginal discomfort, mood swings, or urinary incontinence. Your hysterectomy will not keep you from experiencing some of these symptoms, unless you are part of the 15 percent of women who have no menopausal signs.

If you only have one ovary, it should be able to compensate for the loss of the other ovary as long as it is functioning properly. However, you should make sure your doctor tracks your ovarian function and performs blood tests to determine if you are menopausal.

Hormone Replacement Therapy

As with prematurely menopausal women whose condition is not related to surgery or cancer treatments, the evidence is strong that estrogen replacement should be given to oophorectomized women. In addition, most doctors feel therapy should continue to the biological age of menopause, 51, at which point a woman can reevaluate whether or not to continue.

It is becoming standard procedure to give oophorectomized women estrogen replacement for six to eight weeks after the surgery to alleviate any discomfort that may be associated with menopausal symptoms. After that, you will have to make a conscious decision about whether or not to remain on estrogen therapy.

On the plus side, it is important to emphasize the protection hormone replacement therapy offers against heart disease and osteoporosis. Because surgically induced menopause seems to increase the risk of heart disease and osteoporosis, this can be an especially important decision.

Nevertheless, according to Dr. Ravnikar, cardiovascular disease and osteoporosis are multifactoral and not just related to estrogen deficiency. "Even if we prescribe these pills to those we best guess we should give them to, in addition to accumulating concrete scientific data on their bone densities, we need to use a multifaceted approach. Doctors should discourage smoking, encourage exercise and good diet, and make sure the patient has enough calcium in her diet."

Like women with premature menopause, young oophorectomized women may also be undertreated with currently recommended doses of hormone replacement therapy. This is often a trial-and-error situation where you may have to work closely with your doctor to get a dosage that works effectively for you.

There is still debate about whether or not to give progesterone, along with estrogen, to women without a uterus. Although progesterone has proven effective in preventing uterine cancer for nonhysterectomized women taking estrogen replacement, it can negate many of the cardiovascular benefits. If you no longer have a uterus, uterine cancer is not a threat. However, doctors also agree that progesterone may protect you from some forms of breast disease and prescribe it with estrogen to hysterectomized women. Taking progesterone comes down to an individual decision to be made by a woman and her doctor based on her specific risk factors (see Chapter 4, "Hormone Replacement Therapy").

Chemically and Radiation-Induced Menopause

Diagnosis for cancer usually comes as a surprise to most people and the time immediately following is filled with critical decision making and doing everything possible to ensure survival. This often includes chemotherapy, radiation, or a combination of the two. Although these procedures are known for their ability to improve prognosis, they may have significant side effects for women, including the onset of menopause.

Chemically induced menopause refers to nonsurgical treatment with drugs for a variety of diseases, the by-product of which brings the functioning of your ovaries to a screeching halt. The same effect often occurs with radiation treatment.

Once the initial cancer crisis has passed, after surgery, chemotherapy, and/or radiation therapy have been performed and the matter of survival is no longer as cloudy, other issues emerge, such as losing your fertility as a result of cancer procedures, having to cope with major sexual problems that never existed before, or suddenly being thrust from the jaws of death into the unknowns of premature and sudden menopause.

Fertility Prospects

Although statistics differ depending on a variety of factors, the prospects for fertility are rather poor after many cancer treatment procedures. Loss of ovarian function is dependent on age, drugs used in chemotherapy—alkylating agents, such as chlorambucil and Cytoxan, and other drugs such as busulfan and vinblastine disrupt ovarian function and halt menstruation—and the doses and duration of chemotherapy. Quite logically, one year of chemotherapy is more likely to halt ovarian function than six months of treatment. Subsequent fertility is also dependent on where the cancer is located. If it is in one of the reproductive organs, like the uterus or ovaries, and that organ has to be removed, infertility results. The type of cancer can play a role, too. Certain types of treatments for cancers, like those for Hodgkin's disease, are kinder to women in terms of fertility than to men.

In most cases, the loss of ovarian function is permanent. In women over age 30, there is an 80 percent chance of losing periods forever. Although ovarian function may resume after a hiatus of four months or more, conception after chemotherapy—even with renewed menstrual cycling—is not often possible. According to a book on this subject, *Coping with Chemotherapy* (Nancy Bruning; Garden City, NY: Dial Press, 1985), "Permanent sterility is most common in patients who receive high-dose long-term chemotherapy, such as for Hodgkin's disease, and less common in low-dose short-term chemo plans such as adjuvant [additional] treatment for breast cancer."

Likewise, radiation therapy can cause loss of menstrual periods, though the outcome is dependent on the dose and whether the reproductive organs are located in the field of radiation. When radiation is directed at the pelvis, virtually all women lose function permanently. As with chemotherapy, age and total treatment dose are other factors that can determine fertility following radiation therapy. Younger women, who have a greater number of eggs to begin with, are more likely to resume normal menstrual periods after treatment than are older women.

For women who undergo combination therapy—chemotherapy and pelvic irradiation or the use of multiple chemotherapeutic agents—the prognosis for future fertility is very poor.

This woman describes what it was like for her to suddenly lose her ability to have a child. Even with a philosophical attitude, she found her situation to be troubling and sad.

Within the last twelve months, I've had maternal feelings that are off the charts. In reality, I know I don't want a child, but suddenly becoming menopausal is like watching an opportunity go right out the door. You want to hold on in some way. You think, maybe before this is all over, you should just have a sampling.

Married woman, 49

Infertility Prevention and Counseling

Until recently, there was very little doctors could do to protect the ovaries during various regimens of treatment for cancer. Fortunately, with time come advances in medical technology, and there are now a variety of options available for preserving your fertility. Some of them are still experimental and others may not be appropriate for your situation, but they do exist and more work is being done in this area every day.

One strategy is to get the ovaries out of the picture. For example, prior to radiation therapy, the ovaries can be moved temporarily—tucked under the bladder in a surgical procedure called *oophoropexy*—to protect them. With this procedure, your risk of ovarian dysfunction is reduced by 40 to 50 percent. Doctors can also modify the radiation technique so that the ovaries are shielded from the damaging rays.

A similar strategy of making the ovaries less vulnerable is often used with chemotherapy patients. By prescribing oral contraceptives, doctors can try to downregulate—suppress the ovaries and hormone functions—and create a quiescent state. It appears that more follicles are preserved this way, but it remains uncertain as to whether your fertility rate will improve. Doctors also try to preserve fertility by avoiding chemotherapeutic agents most associated with subsequent loss of ovarian function, namely, the alkylating drugs.

More recently, women have been given the opportunity to bank their ova prior to therapy (see the section on late pregnancy in this chapter for more information). Although this sounds like a great idea, there are still some unresolved problems. The technique is new, and experience is limited. More importantly, time is a critical factor in this procedure. Weeks and sometimes months are needed to stimulate follicles and harvest enough eggs, and most cancer patients do not have enough time to do this.

Another option is donor eggs (ova from another woman), which can be used if you cannot produce your own or are concerned about their quality after a cancer procedure. Although there is no evidence that chemotherapy increases the number of abnormal births, doctors say chemotherapy-related abnormalities would not show up in the next generation anyway, but in two or three generations later.

Even with these potential safeguards against infertility, counseling women undergoing chemotherapy or radiation treatment about possible problems with fertility is standard procedure. However, depending on a doctor's individual style and the hospital where the procedures are performed, the quality of counseling can vary enormously. This can be a complex issue, and it is important to have the most up-to-date advice available. Make certain you get thorough answers to your questions and, if necessary, do not hesitate to seek out other sources of help and information.

Sudden Menopause

Similar to hysterectomy, menopause after chemically induced loss of ovarian function is sudden, and indicators may be slightly greater in intensity than for other women. Research indicates that women recovering from breast, uterine, or ovarian cancers often have more severe menopausal signs. However, the varying degree of severity is difficult to quantify because of the wide range of individual experiences occurring in all women at menopause. Hot flashes, vaginal dryness, and mood swings are common signs of menopause at any age, but with chemically induced menopause, they will often appear suddenly and almost overnight. To make matters worse, they are often combined with the aftereffects of surgery, chemotherapy, or radiation.

Sexual Problems

There are certainly sexual issues associated with chemotherapy and radiation treatment, and most of them stem from a temporary loss of libido, fear of active sex during an uncomfortable recovery period, and vaginal dryness. In some cases, patients are not even informed that their sex lives will be affected by their medical procedures, and the subsequent sexual difficulties can come as a real shock, as they did for this woman.

> I was in the hospital for seven weeks. People told me I might get cataracts, for sure I would lose my hair, and that I had a one in 19 chance of getting lung cancer, but nobody bothered to tell me that they would be screwing up my sex life.
>
> Married mother, 48

One of the critical issues is to acknowledge these problems exist. Many women are still embarrassed about discussing sex, even after living through a battery of invasive procedures to treat disease. There is no reason to think your sex life has to end because of chemotherapy or radiation treatment. Open lines of communication with your partner, seek out counseling from a sex therapist, and, most of all, do not get discouraged. Specific techniques for getting your sex life back on track are discussed in detail in Chapter 7, "Sex."

After my cancer treatment, I decided to interview several gynecologists in order to have one closer to my home for follow-up visits. On the wall of one of the prospective doctors was a big sign saying Infertility Specialist. So I walked in and said to the doctor, "Let's get something straight. I do not need another child and am not interested in infertility . . . I am here because of vaginal dryness. I am here because I had a bone marrow transplant and my sex life has gone to hell in a hand basket."

Then we talked a little about my sex life, or lack of one. He said, "How often are you having sex?" I said, "Maybe once a month." He replied, "How often would you like to have sex?" Easily, I said, "How about once a day!" When talking about my hormone dosage, I mentioned that it was higher than normal. He said, "There's no reason to cut you back to 0.6 milligram of estrogen from 0.9 milligram. If you are comfortable at 0.9 and you're getting more vaginal dryness at 0.6 milligram, you should stay at 0.9."

This doctor is phenomenal! He's funny and bright and treats you like a human and not like some jerk who just got off the boat. He doesn't look at me as some crazy woman going through menopause who gets herself in a flap and never knows if she's doing the right thing. This man is a normal, wonderful, sympathetic person. And he understands my special issues.

Married mother, 50

Emotional Fallout

It is well known that many women who have been treated for cancer suffer from a persistent psychic trauma that their body has failed them. What is not as easily understood is the feelings a woman in this situation may harbor about early menopause, loss of fertility, and sexual dysfunction. The cessation of menstruation can be yet another reminder of bodily failure and betrayal. The loss of fertility in a cancer patient puts her at a disadvantage in terms of the latest reproductive technologies and can be the source of anxiety, discomfort, and emotional suffering. Sexual dysfunction can prevent you from having the affection, warmth, and sense of acceptance so necessary for a long-term recovery.

Counseling can be helpful, but frequently it does not give the patient enough detailed information for her to properly set expectations. Take the story of a 47-year-old woman who experienced chemotherapy-induced menopause after treatment for breast cancer. She had heavy bleeding, violent hot flashes, nausea, anorexia, joint pains, cystitis, vaginal sores, and painful spots on her face. Some symptoms were apparently side effects of the cancer treatment; some were related to sudden premature menopause. She had been counseled about menopause but still found herself disoriented and frustrated about going through "two of the major physical events of my life at once." Because her doctors were unaware of her feelings and overloaded with work, she had to figure out which symptoms were related to which events largely on her own. This woman and those she found having a similar experience felt angry about the inadequate level of support and counseling.

> We would have been able to handle the stress of menopause better if we had known more about what to expect. We agreed that someone ought to prepare some supportive educational materials for women who are about to be whisked unsuspecting into menopause via chemotherapy.
>
> —A Friend Indeed,
> November 1990

Treatment with Estrogen Replacement Therapy

So why not just take estrogen replacement therapy and avoid sudden menopause entirely? Unfortunately, the type of cancer often dictates whether or not you are a candidate for estrogen replacement. For example, women with estrogen-dependent cancer—most notably breast cancer growth, which is stimulated by estrogen in 60 to 70 percent of all cases—are usually poor prospects.

Like most matters associated with hormone replacement therapy, this remains a controversial issue. Dr. William Hoskins, a gynecologic oncologist at Memorial Sloan-Kettering Cancer Center, says, "In general, no, we don't give estrogen replacement therapy to women who have had breast cancer. But the issue of ERT in breast cancer patients hasn't really been studied."

In a recent *New York Times* article, Dr. William L. McGuire, a cancer expert at the Texas Health Science Center in San Antonio, said, "A woman whose [breast] cancer had these estrogen receptors may not want to take the hormone. But a woman whose tumor did not have estrogen receptors and whose cancer was thought unlikely to recur might want to take estrogen."

In the same article, Dr. Veronica Ravnikar, director of Reproductive Endocrinology, Fertility, Menopause at the University of Massachusetts Medical Center, said that she often sees cancer patients who are feeling desperate about menopausal symptoms. "I've had situations where these patients come in and say: 'I don't care if I do have a recurrence. I have these hot flashes so bad I can't sleep.' [All I can do] is give these patients the limited information [available] so that they can weigh the risks and make a choice."

Still, doctors are often reluctant to recommend estrogen to women who have had breast cancer because of fears of malpractice. They just do not have enough answers about estrogen and its likelihood of stimulating cancer growth.

Many women who have had breast cancer or have a family history of it may make the decision about whether to take estrogen replacement therapy based on their personal "fear" meter—whether they are more afraid of cancer or of osteoporosis and heart disease. This woman's fear of her cancer recurring far outweighed any benefits that might come from taking hormone replacement therapy.

I won't take hormone replacement therapy because of my breast cancer. The night sweats are bad enough. I don't need to add to my sleeplessness by staying up all night wondering about what my odds would be for getting cancer again if I was on ERT. So I do other things to combat the effects of menopause. I make myself stay up as late as I can so that I'm exhausted when my head hits the pillow and less likely to be awakened by a hot flash. I've given up caffeine, cut way back on wine with dinner, and try to keep up with my exercise routine, not only for bone density reasons, but to help with my sleeping as well. It's not a perfect solution, but it's the best I can do right now.

Single mother, 49

Women in premature menopause as a result of chemotherapy may be even more likely than women who go through menopause naturally to develop heart disease or osteoporosis. It comes down to a numbers game. If you start menopause earlier, you will have more years ahead of you when your ovaries are not producing sufficient estrogen to up your risk of osteoporosis and heart disease.

Other forms of cancer occurring in reproductive organs do not necessarily rule out estrogen replacement therapy. Dr. Bruce Patsner, a gynecologic oncologist practicing in Redbank, New Jersey, says, "Generally speaking, patients who have cervical, vulvar, vaginal, or even most types of ovarian cancer can be put on estrogen replacement therapy."

There definitely is debate over the use of estrogen replacement therapy after endometrial (uterine) cancer, however. Some experts say it should not be used at all, some say you can use it right away, and some say you should wait about a year. Gynecologic oncologists are looking closely at this issue in order to get some clear answers.

In any case, if you opt for estrogen replacement therapy, it is critical that you track your health carefully. This means regular mammograms and frequent exams if you have had breast cancer. You should also have your cholesterol levels and bone density closely monitored. If you still have a uterus, it is important to take progesterone with estrogen to guard against uterine cancer (see Chapter 4, "Hormone Replacement Therapy"). Although both naturally and chemically induced menopausal women experience vaginal dryness in the same way, women have a variable response to hormone replacement therapy. Data suggest that standard doses of hormone replacement therapy may not be adequate for vaginal dryness experienced after chemotherapy. Be aware of this and work patiently with your doctor to come up with a dosage that works for you.

You may even have to be more proactive than that if your experience is similar to that of this woman, who was recovering from a bone marrow transplant.

I have discovered that very few oncologists know the first thing about estrogen replacement therapy. What's more, it is rare when one of them actually gives you advice when you're going through chemotherapy or radiation that estrogen therapy is probably going to be necessary. On my last day in the hospital, a group of doctors asked me what I was looking forward to the most. And I said, sleeping with my husband. Not one person, not a doctor or a nurse, said, "Excuse me, have we taken care of this lady's estrogen level?" Not one medical person said, "Make sure you see someone in endocrinology about your estrogen level." Not one woman thought to say to me, "Do you realize that vaginal dryness means pain during sex?"

Married mother, 50

Tamoxifen for Women with Breast Cancer

Tamoxifen, sold under the trade name Nolvadex, is an oral drug that blocks the effects of estrogen and is often referred to as an antiestrogen drug. For the past twenty years, it has been used to treat advanced breast cancer, because it slows or stops the growth of breast cancer cells. More recently, according to the National Cancer Institute, it is being used, with great success, as an adjuvant, or additional, therapy following primary treatment for early-stage breast cancer. Studies are also being conducted to test tamoxifen's effectiveness in treating other types of cancer such as melanoma, endometrial cancer, and certain leukemias.

As adjuvant therapy, tamoxifen reduces the recurrence of breast cancer, prevents the development of new cancers in the opposite breast, and improves survival. Tamoxifen even appears to work in breast cancer tumors that are not dependent on estrogen, leading National Cancer Institute investigator Dr. Andrew Dorr to remark, "The drug probably has other mechanisms of action. It may be a tumor suppressor in and of itself." It has also been found that tamoxifen's cancer-fighting benefits persist long after—at least ten years—treatment stops.

Postmenopausal women have been the subject of most of the studies on tamoxifen. Consequently, its benefits and risks in premenopausal women are less well known. According to an article in the *Journal of Clinical Oncology*, "Tamoxifen offers a favorable therapeutic alternative for premenopausal women with estrogen-receptor-positive metastatic breast cancer who wish to avoid surgical or radiation castration."

The full picture on tamoxifen can be a little confusing. It acts against the effects of estrogen in breast tissue, thereby preventing cancer. However, it also acts just like estrogen in other parts of the body. This means it provides many of the same benefits as estrogen replacement therapy, such as positively affecting blood cholesterol and lowering cardiovascular disease risk, while at the same time slowing bone loss and offering protection against osteoporosis. So for postmenopausal women who cannot take estrogen replacement therapy because of breast cancer, tamoxifen may be a reasonable alternative.

However, the tamoxifen data are still not clear for younger women, especially in terms of its benefit on bone loss after premature menopause. Dr. Daiva Bajorunas, an endocrinologist at Memorial Sloan-Kettering Cancer Center, says, "The evidence is pretty convincing that in postmenopausal women with breast cancer, tamoxifen is protective. But we still don't know if it is as protective as estrogen replacement therapy. The tougher question is for a woman who is 36, has early-stage breast disease, receives adjuvant chemotherapy, and loses her period at 37. We don't know if tamoxifen is as protective as her not losing her periods. Some, but not very good, data show tamoxifen is not protective in younger women, but few studies have been done on younger women overall."

Lack of information on tamoxifen and its experimental nature, combined with a shaky recovery from chemotherapy, led this woman to pass on the option of taking this drug. This dilemma is a common one for many cancer patients.

I've had Hodgkin's disease and after major surgery, chemotherapy, and radiation treatment went through instant menopause as well. The oncologist wanted to put me on hormones, but my regular doctor and an endocrinologist advised against it. My bone density is low and my biggest concern is around osteoporosis at this point. I've looked into taking tamoxifen, but it's too experimental and I don't want to be a guinea pig. Once you go through chemotherapy, I don't think your body is ever the same.

Single mother, 55

One specific area where the effects of tamoxifen differ from estrogen replacement therapy is in abating hot flashes. It just does not help at all. In fact, one of the side effects of tamoxifen, experienced by 4 to 5 percent of all women taking the drug, is hot flashes. This small group of women may also suffer from a variety of side effects, some of which are similar to those associated with menopause. These effects can include nausea, vomiting, and weight gain; less common are bone pain, changes in menstrual periods, vaginal discharge or bleeding, headache, genital itching, and skin rash or dryness. Often the side effects disappear as your body adjusts to treatment. Other side effects can include depression, noted in only 1 percent of postmenopausal women using tamoxifen as adjuvant therapy; data from clinical trials suggest a small risk of blood clots equivalent to the risk in women taking birth control pills or estrogen replacement therapy. Fortunately, 95 percent of women taking tamoxifen do so successfully without side effects.

Even with tamoxifen's high level of acceptability, big questions remain about tamoxifen and the risks of endometrial and liver cancer. According to the National Cancer Institute,

> Results from several large clinical trials suggest that women taking the usual dose of tamoxifen (20 mg/day) have an increased risk of cancer of the lining of the uterus (endometrial cancer). The risk of endometrial cancer is about doubled by tamoxifen, an increase similar to that associated with estrogen replacement therapy in postmenopausal women. There has also been some concern that tamoxifen may cause liver cancer. In one adjuvant trial, liver tumors were reported in 2 of 931 breast cancer patients receiving a high dose (40 mg/day) of tamoxifen. In these cases, it is not known whether the liver tumors were caused by the drug or were the result of breast cancer that had spread to the liver. In six other trials using 20 mg of tamoxifen daily as adjuvant therapy, no liver cancers have been reported.

A large-scale study is now under way to see if tamoxifen can prevent breast cancer in high-risk women. The National Cancer Institute plans to study 16,000 women, randomly assigning half to tamoxifen and half to a placebo, for five years. Eligible candidates for study are women 60 and older, because they have the highest risk of breast cancer, and women 35 to 59 who have a family history of the disease or a personal medical history of breast lumps, which increases their risk of breast cancer to that of a 60-year-old woman. Opponents of the study are concerned about testing this potent, far from benign, drug in healthy women.

What about the use of tamoxifen as an alternative to estrogen replacement therapy? It is highly unlikely that doctors will prescribe it for most women. Dr. Ravnikar says, "Tamoxifen isn't something you can prescribe as an estrogen alternative. Besides, tamoxifen doesn't seem to have a good clinical effect on hot flashes. It may have some effect on bone and may actually preserve bone mass. But other than that, it really isn't a clear substitute for estrogen. For the breast cancer patient who may not be able to go on hormones, it may be a valid option. But to use it in someone who doesn't have breast cancer, just because they don't want to take estrogen, doesn't seem appropriate."

From a regulatory standpoint, tamoxifen is restricted in its approval. There are physicians who might prescribe it for women who do not want to take estrogen and who have a family member with a history of breast cancer, but currently it is only approved for women with a history of breast cancer to use prophylactically.

Uterine Fibroids

One of the popular reasons for hysterectomy, uterine fibroids seem to be most prevalent among perimenopausal women. Approximately 25 percent of all women over 35 have them. This is hardly a comforting thought, except that 99 percent of all fibroids are benign and most do not require treatment.

Usually attached to the uterine wall, fibroids are made up of muscle and fibrous connective tissue and require estrogen for their growth. Why they occur is still unknown, but they commonly shrink or disappear after menopause, when estrogen supply is at a low ebb. Many women with fibroids learn about their existence only from a watchful physician, whereas others may be plagued with various side effects. Fibroids have been known to cause abnormal or heavy menstrual bleeding, enlargement of the abdomen, and general pain and discomfort. Larger fibroids may grow in such a way as to put pressure on the bladder, ureter, or rectum, in which case surgery is usually necessary.

Taking a conservative approach, this woman hopes she will be able to avoid surgery completely.

I've had fibroids since I was 35, and hysterectomy has been strongly suggested. For lots of reasons, I don't want to have one unless it's absolutely necessary. Recently I've found a new doctor who is very supportive about waiting it out and avoiding surgery. I'm actually looking forward to menopause at this point because there's a strong possibility that when it happens, my fibroids will shrink down to nothing. At least, that's what I'm hoping for.

Married woman, 53

There are several ways to deal with fibroids, and if you are close to menopause, most doctors recommend waiting and watching carefully. However, if you fall into the smaller group of women with serious fibroid problems or are too young to wait it out, there are a few alternatives to hysterectomy worth considering.

- *Myomectomy*, like hysterectomy, is still considered major surgery and is performed under general anesthesia. The benefit of this option is that fibroids of almost any size and number can be eradicated without removing your uterus, thus allowing you to have children if you so desire. Because myomectomy may entail significant blood loss, often requiring transfusions, many physicians still prefer hysterectomy.
- A *hysteroscope–resectoscope* is used in a relatively new procedure done on an outpatient basis. The instrument is inserted into your uterus via the vagina and can remove small fibroids. This procedure only takes about thirty minutes, and recovery time is minimal, especially as compared to the four to six weeks associated with hysterectomy. Because of its recent discovery, this procedure is often available only at medical centers in large cities: however, your doctor can arrange for you to have this done if you are willing to travel.
- *Lupron* is a drug used to shrink fibroids, which works by suppressing your production of estrogen. Its major benefit is in preoperative use: If your fibroid is smaller, you will lose less blood and have a quicker recovery. Lupron is available by injection; without surgery it will only provide temporary relief by shrinking fibroids. Because it suppresses estrogen, its side effects include hot flashes, vaginal dryness, and bone loss.

- *RU-486*, the French abortion pill, also shrinks fibroids but works differently by suppressing progesterone, which is also thought to contribute to fibroid growth. Again, it is most effectively used preoperatively. As of this writing, RU-486 is still not available in the United States.
- *Myoma coagulation* is a brand-new strategy pioneered by Dr. Herbert Goldfarb, director of the department of gynecology at Montclair Community Hospital in New Jersey. It works by shrinking the fibroid and then cutting off its blood supply, all done handily in an outpatient procedure with the aid of Lupron and a laparoscope, a combination viewer and laser instrument. This is a promising alternative for women with fibroids less than ten centimeters in size. It is not recommended for women who still want to have children because of its unknown effect on fertility.

This woman was fortunate enough to be able to endure her fibroids, wait it out, and benefit from the onset of menopause. Her fibroids simply shrank and disappeared.

By the time I reached 47, I began to have a lot of heavy bleeding and was diagnosed as having fibroids. I almost had to have a hysterectomy at 48—I would start my period and it would last for months, or I would have four or five days of bleeding, stop for a few days, and then have two or three more days of bleeding, and so on. I mean it was a constant battle and not much fun. I got very thin and anemic, and my doctor strongly recommended a hysterectomy. I battled like crazy not to have one, and by some incredible miracle, at 49 I began to bleed less. At 50, the bleeding stopped altogether. So, I'm one of the lucky people who survived fibroids without a hysterectomy.

Married mother, 58

Although fibroids require estrogen to grow, they are typically not affected by standard doses of hormone replacement therapy. However, if you have fibroids and opt for hormone replacement therapy, your doctor will probably insist on careful and frequent monitoring of your condition. In this situation, you will still have to weigh the long-term benefits of hormone replacement therapy against the emotional stress of dealing with benign fibroid tumors.

Late Pregnancy

> My gorgeous girl came from a 41-year-old egg.
> —Actress Glenn Close
> on the birth of her daughter, Annie

Baby boomers are a savvy, take-charge bunch, and their quest for everything the world has to offer has driven them to pursue academics, careers, financial goals, life, multiple partners, marriage, and divorce. Now the first wave of baby boomers, in their 40s, is on the brink of menopause. Along the way, many of these women may have forgotten, neglected, or postponed childbirth, remaining childless in their prime reproductive years.

Now the group who wanted to have it all is making the late baby business boom. Many women in their late 30s and early 40s have decided to get off the career track and turn their attention to baby making.

Hollywood is a good example of the popularity of this trend: Ann Jillian had a baby boy at 41 after breast cancer, Candice Bergen had her first child at 39, Bette Midler did it at 40, Glenn Close and Mia Farrow had children at 41, Cheryl Tiegs had her first at 43, Susan Sarandon had her third at 42, Diana Ross started a second family at 43, Goldie Hawn and Sigourney Weaver did it at 40. Connie Chung, now in her 40s, cut back on her grueling broadcast schedule in a last-gasp attempt to have a baby before menopause. Even fictional mom Murphy Brown did it in her 40s—much to the chagrin of former Vice President Dan Quayle.

The real-life women are not far behind. Newspaper headlines are chock-full of stories of women who have gone through high-tech in vitro fertilization procedures, received donor eggs, stored eggs or embryos for future use—even a woman who, at age 42, gave birth to her own grandchildren: Her daughter, born without a uterus, had eggs removed from her ovaries, fertilized outside her body by her husband's sperm, and then implanted in her mother's womb. The result: twins!

Despite the odds, and there are many, today's women are trying to push the envelope of time and fertility. Late pregnancies are up by 37 percent after a downward trend since the peak of 1975. Through new in vitro fertilization techniques, it is even possible for women past menopause to have babies.

Fertility specialist Dr. Mark Sauer of the University of Southern California has developed techniques enabling older women, even menopausal women, to achieve pregnancy. Dr. Sauer attributes some of this success to an attitude and spirit many of these former 1960s activist women still maintain. Now in their late 40s, they are the same group of women who challenged conventional thinking back when they were teenagers. According to Dr. Sauer, "Menopause is another opportunity to raise the gauntlet and question the conventional wisdom that says: 'You're too old to have a baby.' They want to do it and they're not to be denied. I've seen a very persistent, aggressive group of women who really want to have children late in life. And they'll spend a great deal of time and money and go through a lot to make it happen."

Fertility and the Numbers
A lack of understanding of just what it takes to get pregnant as you grow older is a major contributing factor to infertility. At 25, your odds of conceiving after one year of trying are 89 percent; after 30, 84 percent; and after 35, 77 percent. By the time you reach 40, the odds drop significantly. So picture a 35-year-old couple who discontinue contraception in an effort to conceive a child. It may be a year before they realize that specialized help might be in order, and depending on the nature of the problem, fertility treatments can take years, thus lowering the odds for success.

In addition to age, gynecological problems like endometriosis and uterine fibroids become more common in women in their late 30s and 40s and can often prevent pregnancy. Your ovulation patterns also change long before menopause occurs. According to the book *Childbearing After 35* (Dr. Francesca C. Fay and Kathy S. Smith; New York: Balsam Press, 1985), "By the time you turn 40, 3 out of 12 cycles may be infertile; this increases to 7 out of 12 by the time you're 46." In addition, the eggs that are left often do not respond normally to fertilization and may not implant correctly in the uterus.

Many doctors refer to two separate ovarian events surrounding menopause: the well-known endocrine menopause, where your periods stop around the age of 51, and the reproductive menopause, which occurs about ten years before your periods stop. It is during this phase of reproductive menopause that women see the first signs of ovarian failure, a gradual process that does not happen overnight. During this time, women who have normal menstrual cycles assume they are fertile and are frequently caught off guard to find their ovaries are not producing well in terms of egg quality or may not be producing any eggs at all.

So when all is said and done, becoming pregnant in your late 30s or 40s is no mean feat. The irony is that pregnancy in women over 40 is frequently unplanned and unwanted and the number of legal abortions is high (see Chapter 7, "Sex").

Older Pregnancy

In addition to carrying a child with a higher risk of birth defects, older pregnant women tend to suffer from hypertension, diabetes, preeclampsia (metabolic disturbance caused by edema and hypertension), and premature labor more than younger women. Miscarriage and obstetrical complications are more common over the age of 35, and cesarean sections are performed more frequently during delivery.

Still, recent studies indicate that even though older women have higher complication rates of pregnancy and delivery, their risk of poor perinatal outcome is not appreciably higher than that of younger mothers.

Why Women Wait

One strong indicator of the difficult outlook for older pregnancy is an increased demand for high-tech pregnancy procedures. Even more interesting are the social and cultural factors that drive women to opt for later pregnancy.

- Women in midlife frequently undergo marital changes. Some get married later in life for the first or even second time and still want a family. These women have the same desire as younger couples to have a family with their new husbands.
- Women who have postponed childbirth for professional career growth run into difficulty conceiving in their late 30s and 40s. Despite being well educated, they find themselves in the dilemma of underestimating biological changes that come with age.
- Women who have raised a family with a husband or on their own just want to do it all over again.

These are common situations and, if anything, the trend seems to be moving toward even older women having children. Dr. Sauer reports, "It used to be that most of the women I did embryo transplantation to were in their 30s. But in the last two or three years, it's been increasingly in women in their middle to late 40s. Now, in the last year, I've seen a shift even toward 50-year-olds."

The World of High-Technology Pregnancy

A good friend once asked me, "Isn't there anything you can do to stop menopause and still have babies? Some drug you can take, some high-tech procedure?" At the time, I said no, but with medical breakthroughs happening all the time, I have had to eat my words. It is definitely possible for a menopausal woman to carry a child to full term.

In a procedure pioneered by Dr. Sauer, a combination of hormones that have the effect of "rejuvenating" the womb are administered to a menopausal woman. Then an embryo, formed from the husband's sperm and a donor egg, is implanted in the uterus. The procedures are fairly successful—about one-third of the women get pregnant—and have changed the lives of several menopausal women who thought they would never be able to have children.

The Effects on Menopause

With all of the extraordinary methods often used to ensure a late pregnancy, it is a relief to know that menopause is not affected. There is no evidence that late pregnancies, multiple pregnancies, or the use of long-term oral contraceptives have any effect on the time of arrival of menopause or on its symptoms.

Dr. Sauer suspects that for women who conceive on their own later in life, their chance of having a later menopause is probably greater. Their ability to conceive is an indication that they still have good ovarian function and that communication between their hypothalamus, pituitary gland, and ovaries is working well.

Similarly, there is no evidence that fertility drugs or procedures have any effect on menopause—making it arrive earlier or later, or causing symptoms to be better or worse.

Chapter Nine

Men and Menopause

Can we talk? I was out for dinner, playing corporate wife, and found myself sitting at a table of five men, all in their late 40s. After we had dispensed with the usual pleasantries and business had been discussed ad nauseam, one of the men turned to me and asked about the subject of my book. When I replied I was writing about menopause, he was a little surprised. Nevertheless, he bravely plunged ahead and asked why I had chosen the subject. By that time, general conversation had come to a screeching halt, and all eyes were focused in my direction. I said it was because I had started menopause two years ago and could not find enough information on the subject. Well, every jaw at the table, except my husband's, of course, dropped. "But you can't be." "You're too young, ha, ha." "Did you say menopause?" "Is it a humorous book?" This articulate group of marketing geniuses was unable to put together a single comprehensible response. And did they ever squirm—all the way through dessert.

I still laugh when I think about that evening and many other casual conversations with men about writing this book. But after spending more time interviewing men, gaining insight from the women who love them, talking to psychologists and researchers, and learning about the male perspective, I have developed a more sympathetic attitude.

What Men Think About Menopause

Most men just do not get it. So much about women has always seemed mysterious and somewhat taboo to them, and when it comes to menopause, they cannot figure out where to begin.

In many ways, men are not to blame. Menopause was rarely part of their education, either at home or in school, and until recently women were reticent to broach the subject with one another, never mind a man. These close-mouthed women are the same ones who marched their husbands to Lamaze childbirth classes in an effort to share the experience and gain help and support from their mate. Most of the time it worked, and you would think with this kind of previous shared intimacy, it would not be difficult to make the leap to having a discussion about menopause, at the very least. However, these kinds of conversations are not occurring, and men are more in the dark than ever about one of the most pivotal experiences in a woman's life.

Furthermore, men do not have a clue about where to begin, as explained by this articulate advertising executive.

> I haven't asked my wife about menopause. I guess we don't talk about it. But what are you supposed to talk about anyway? If somebody has an allergy, do you sit down and talk about it: "Hi, how's your allergy? I notice your nose has been running a lot." I don't know the currency of a conversation about menopause. I don't know when menopause starts or stops or even what happens afterward. It's just something I haven't thought that much about. It doesn't seem to be impeding our relationship in any way—so it's not really an issue.
>
> Married father, 57

Assuming you are one of the few women who do discuss menopause with your mate, you may have felt you were not being heard, and for good reason. Even when confronted with the facts about menopause, men find it difficult to relate. They have no experience in their lives close to what occurs during menopause and often cannot identify with what is happening to you. Truth be told, men are not likely to pay much attention unless your menopausal experience begins to affect them directly, such as with interrupted sleep because of your hot flashes or less frequent sex as a result of vaginal dryness.

Another factor that can show up as indifference in your mate is his own obsession with what is happening in his life. Unfortunately, menopause usually coincides with the time men are focused on their own midlife issues. They are often preoccupied with problems at work, career path, signs of their physical decline, and perhaps the unknowns of aging. And you want them to take a quiet minute and understand all about menopause?

Nevertheless, according to a recent Gallup survey of 705 men married to women aged 40 to 60, two-thirds of them were concerned about the effects of menopause on their wives. This is a fairly high percentage, leading one to believe that men really do care. When a man is confronted with the subject of menopause, perhaps some of his lack of response is based more on ignorance, embarrassment, and a fear of looking foolish. Later in this chapter, you will find ways to discuss menopause with your mate and avoid this seeming indifference. It would be wonderful to have the kind of support and understanding shown by this man who has been married to the same woman for twenty-two years.

I think menopause is a major event in my wife's life, like a passage. There are a lot of different things that go on. Look at the statement it makes. You're no longer able to bear children; you're getting older. And from the psychological standpoint, it is like a man's midlife crisis. Menopause means you're that much closer to old age, to death. It's a time when you're more likely to lose your parents, or they'll become frail and need a great deal of care. It is a natural time for a woman to say to herself consciously or sub-consciously, What am I doing here? What am I doing with my life? Is this really what I want . . . with my husband, with my family? It's a moment to reflect and say, Where did I go wrong? Or right? How did it come to this?

                                                    Married father, 54

What Men Know About Menopause

If you put a group of men and women in a room and gave them a quick quiz on the basics of menopause, the women would perform from above average to poor and almost all of the men would flunk. This is hardly a surprise. Until recently, there has not been a lot of readily available information on the subject, and none of it has been geared toward men.

Without much knowledge, men have still formed opinions about menopause. They seem to know little, if anything, about hot flashes, vaginal dryness, or other physical indicators. They do, however, focus on the negative impact of menopause on women's emotions. Whether this is sparked by a memory of a cranky middle-aged mother or day-to-day experiences with a mate is unclear. According to a recent poll of men employed at a large midwestern university—most of whom were educated professionals with at least one child—45 percent expressed a belief that most women are depressed about menopause and 37 percent said depression was the most common change-of-life complaint. Even this executive, who had a handle on the subject, showed a bias toward the emotional side of the issue.

First of all, I don't know a lot. I think it happens around middle age, late 40s or early 50s. It's a physiological thing that has to do with hormonal changes and it's accompanied by mood swings. You hear these horrible stories about how grumpy women get and how out of sorts they become. Basically, it's a transition women go through when their periods stop and their hormones change. After that, they hopefully recover and come back to what we would call a normal state, somewhat similar to before, or perhaps move into a changed state. During this time, there are some hormone supplements they can take to make the transition easier. And that's about it.

Single father, 52

Many men also feel it is not their place to be knowledgeable about menopause. To them, it is a woman's issue best dealt with by other women. In other words, leave men out.

Menopause is such a specific problem that men have no knowledge of it. It would be like asking a guy for his advice on sanitary napkins. It's something he doesn't know anything about. Most men don't—even the experts, the doctors, don't know what's going on.

Married father, 56

However, some men would truly welcome a crash course on menopause as long as it did not take up too much time and focused on aspects relevant to them. Other men even indicated a desire to have a list of menopause no-no's to help guide them through social and professional situations with menopausal women. It sounds like a good idea, but you can bet that these same men are not about to pick up a book on menopause or attend a hospital-sponsored symposium usually targeted to women. It is doubtful that they would even read a magazine article on menopause.

There's not much I need to know about menopause—I've read and heard enough. I certainly don't need the clinical details. I know that in some cases it can cause pretty severe psychological problems and sometimes physical problems. I'm aware of the sexual impact, the lessening of desire and lack of lubrication. And I'm sensitive to the fact that menopause is a statement that says, "You're getting old, kid. You can't make babies anymore, and even though you may think that's wonderful, it's still a cross to bear. It sets you apart from all the younger women out there." It can come at a moment of potential midlife crisis where you question what life is all about: Did I accomplish what I set out to do?

So I'm aware of all those things. Do I have to know much more? I hope not. To sit down and read books—forget it.

Married father, 53

Do not despair: There is a handy seven-point primer in Appendix 1 written specifically for men. It just might do the trick for your mate.

How Men Feel About Menopausal Women

When all is said and done—you have dealt with hot flashes, vaginal dryness, mood swings, incontinence—postmenopausal sex appeal remains the issue of the hour. Yes, women are concerned about the threats of osteoporosis and heart disease, but what festers in the back of most of their minds is whether or not they will maintain their attractiveness as women. This anxiety is manifested in questions like

Will men think I'm an old woman?
What about wrinkles and a little bit extra around my hips?
Will I still be attractive to men?
How can I compete with a 30-year-old?
It's great not to worry about getting pregnant, but does that mean I'm less appealing . . . all used up?
Is this the end of admiring glances and a whistle every now and then?

As you might expect, women are their own harshest critics, and their perception of what men find attractive is often inaccurate. The good news is that men are far more forgiving of physical changes than you might imagine. And some of them, like the following man, look beyond the physical to find magnetism in a mate.

If you equate sex appeal with physical appearance and perfection, then you're doomed. I could be shown a pile of photographs of women and, without knowing anything about them, be able to discriminate who turns me on. But that's not what sex appeal is all about. It has more to do with bearing and carriage and manner and self-image. I think the women who are comfortable with themselves show it in an obvious way, and that is very sexually appealing.

Married father, 52

Sex appeal is a rather amorphous concept, and everyone seems to have an opinion. According to Madison Avenue, it is best represented by some nubile young thing, half-dressed, modeling blue jeans or playing volleyball on the beach. Although companies like Lee are now cutting looser jeans called Easy Riders to accommodate fuller thighs and thicker waists, the image of a bone-thin beauty in her late 20s with perfect hair, skin, eyes, and teeth is still the ideal. Americans are obsessed with youth, and the jury is still out as to whether the enticing revenues from middle-aged baby boomer spending will be enough to reshape the image and cause a reevaluation of the worth of older people. Maybe it will happen, but certainly not within the next five or ten years. This means midlife women will have to strike out on their own and create a new model representing vitality, self-confidence, and allure.

There are also men around who believe women are born with sex appeal, sort of like a genetic gift—either you have it or you don't.

I think that there are some women who will always be sexy, regardless of what's succumbing to gravity and what isn't. I mean, they're just sexy people. They feel sexy, they radiate that kind of thing. I think a man picks up on that and would find it to be a turn-on.

Single man, 57

According to some men, if you are among these lucky women, menopause and midlife will not play a big role in your ability to turn heads.

Men talk a good game and their continual ogling of sweet young things is enough to give any woman second thoughts about her looks. However, men are also concerned about their own appearance as they get older. Before the women's revolution, men could easily trade their power and money for a woman's beauty. Now that today's independent women have pursued serious careers and gained power and money of their own, the equation has changed. In an editorial in the July 1992 issue of M Magazine titled "The Changing American Male," editor Clay Felker calls a spade a spade. "Now we are going through a change in the balance of power and men are finding they have to rely increasingly on their looks. Even the raiders of the 1980s, who dumped their old first marriages for new 'trophy' wives, have slimmed down and done their best to look attractive."

So while you may be having a personal crisis over whether or not you are still appealing, your mate may be coping with appearance demons of his own. More and more men are being viewed as sex objects by women, even midlife and older women, and men are finally figuring out the score. They now spend more than $55 million a year on skin care products alone, up from $25 million a decade ago. Men no longer settle for turning gray gracefully and instead keep appointments for eyelash tints, scalp treatments, massages, and cosmetic surgery. This kind of reaction is not limited to the California crowd either. George Bush is known to have a manicure every twelve days and a facial almost as often.

In an effort to keep it all in perspective, one man confessed the following:

> I find my wife as sexually attractive to me as when I first met her. She still excites me—I can't keep my hands off her. Sure I notice that her stomach isn't as toned up as it was, and then once in a while I look in the mirror and realize mine isn't either. Why should aging be any different for women than men?
>
> Married father, 54

Finally, there is a group of men who find older women more attractive. No, this is not a small, spaced-out cult. Men who are not focused on the superficial and have grown in mind and attitude value women their own age. There is also a growing number of younger men who have recently discovered the benefits of a relationship with an older woman. More peace, less self-doubt, wisdom, experience, and a well-developed sense of humor are just a few of the attractions. A Chicago lawyer stated the case quite well.

> I think sex appeal is tied up in your perspective of women in general. From almost every conceivable point of view, women certainly are more interesting as they get older, not less. I think it's always wonderful to look at someone my daughter's age who is beautiful, but I'm not so sure I'd want to marry one of them.
>
> Married father, 57

Changes for Men at Midlife

Women do have the harder row to hoe when it comes to midlife changes, but men do not get off scot-free. After years of work-hard-make-money-get-ahead activity, many men find themselves plagued by self-doubt, depression, and an overwhelming sense of lassitude sometime in their 40s or early 50s. Not much later, the majority of them experience diminished physical capacity, both in terms of sexual performance and overall muscular range and stamina. You may not hear much about these phenomena now, but with the enormous marketing potential represented by millions of aging baby boomers, these physical changes will be making headline news before long. According to Dr. John B. McKinlay, an epidemiologist at Boston University who has studied aging in both men and women, "There's a very strong interest in treating aging men for profit, just as there is for menopausal women."

Changes for men at midlife fall into two basic categories: the psychological, often called *male midlife crisis*, and the physical, euphemistically referred to as male menopause. Just as in women, these changes are real and not a figment of someone's imagination. You have only to listen to this divorce attorney's viewpoint, based on his experience with numerous crisis-plagued men, to be convinced.

Midlife crisis definitely exists. I think it's based on a realization that you only have a certain number of years left in your life and you've loaded yourself with responsibilities that you just can't handle, like a wife who may or may not be satisfactory, but at any rate, you think you can do better. It's almost a reversion to an adolescent attitude—you want to get rid of all your responsibilities and at least, in your own mind, enjoy life in a selfish, self-centered way. And most of the time this is done with no regard to the ramifications of leaving a wife and perhaps children. Men in midlife crisis are dissatisfied with their status and instead of turning their energies toward improving their existing situation, they think things will be better elsewhere, which they usually are not. It's a "grass is greener" type of complex.

Married father, 55

Given the widespread proliferation of midlife crisis, it is worthwhile to take a few minutes to get up to speed on men's issues. By understanding the male side of the midlife equation, women will be well positioned to pave the way toward more fulfilling communication with the opposite sex. Yes, the ball is being hit back into your court, but you, as a woman, are more likely to become informed and make the effort to reach out and change things for the better.

Male Midlife Crisis

One of the positive things about getting older is that sometime in your 40s you stop caring quite as much about certain things that used to be major focal points in your daily life. Maybe it happens because they just are not important anymore in the overall scope. Or it may be that you know these former objects of desire are not realistically within your reach. Either way, you know with certainty that the picture has changed. For some this can be a liberating experience, like being let off the hook, but for others, this can spell disaster.

It is a well-known fact that a man's identity revolves around his potency and strength as well as his success at work and in society. Yet, once a man hits 45, this view of manhood becomes threatened. It is one thing for a middle-aged man to lose a tennis match to his son and quite another to walk into work in the morning and suddenly realize he is never going to be promoted to senior vice president. Men at this age definitely experience significant personal transition, a heightened awareness of themselves, or male midlife crisis.

> *Men and women just have different DNA. A woman's going through menopause and no longer being able to have children is just not traumatic for a man. He's more affected by whether he can fight and play and compete. And when you start to lose that ability, it's a major crisis, whether you're 40, 45, or 50. It's like hot flashes to a man. You say to yourself, "What's happening? I'm no longer that 40ish guy . . . I'm now a 50ish guy." These are very real feelings, maybe similar to how a woman reacts to menopause.*
>
> Married father, 58

A variety of factors influence a man's emotional state at midlife, some of which are shared by women—dealing with teenage children or with a home left empty by their later departure and aging parents who may be sick or dying. At this age, a man often faces the fact that his job has become more limited in terms of future options or that he may not always have a job as a measure of his worth. A successful businessman talked about work as the ultimate life game and said,

> *What I'm really concerned about as I get older has to do with work, about stopping the game. You don't want to not play well; you just want to keep playing. It's great fun to start at the bottom and come up and finish at the top. And when you're at the top, you just want to start all over again. You know, like a kid—I don't*

*want to go to bed, just one more game, just one more show, just
one more. That's what it's all about.*

Married father, 55

According to psychologists, lack of change as well as not
being the center of attention may also depress a man at this time.
No longer is he in the limelight at key events such as weddings,
births, first homes, or outstanding promotions.

Any of these factors can cause a man to feel an enormous
sense of regret: regret that he has not accomplished more or
made enough money or had enough sex or spent more time with
his kids. Men also worry about their ability to continue in their
self-declared role as provider, especially when honestly assessing
their long-term financial prospects.

*I find I'm more aware of the what-ifs, especially when it comes to
my career. I mean, I'm more financially secure than 99.9 percent
of the population, and yet, I find myself thinking sometimes it's
not enough. What if suddenly the business went bad. I see it
happening all around me. I'd have to eat into principal—holy
smokes, I can't even afford to live on the interest I'd earn off the
principal, and I've got plenty of principal. Could it all evaporate?
You always like to think, If I have to do it all over again and
start from scratch, I could. But who the hell wants to?*

Married father, 58

Add to these emotional issues the general effects of aging and
you can wind up with the picture of a man who will do almost
anything to stay young. Talk about escapism. That is just what
happens when a middle-aged man trades in his wife and family
for a younger model. Does a woman's menopause have an effect
on this kind of thinking? Only if you are talking about the type
of man who is naturally uncomfortable in his own skin; then
perhaps his wife's menopause, perceived as a glaring reminder of
his own aging process, is enough to put him over the top.

Older men with younger women is not a new concept, nor
are the factors that bring on this behavior. It has great appeal for

almost all men, but fortunately only a few feel required to act on it.

> I don't think men run around with younger women because they are attractive. It's more the fact that they make men feel younger. I know a lot of men who do it. I don't know that they like those women they're involved with very much—it's more what being with younger women does for them, how it makes them feel. It's a very selfish kind of pursuit.
>
> Married father, 56

Putting morality to one side, most men would love to be seen with a younger woman. In addition to making them feel younger, it raises their image and stature with other men in the great male competitive game of life. After a divorce and before his second marriage to another woman his own age, this man was free to romp, dated several significantly younger women, and loved every minute of it. However, he also was aware of the psychology behind his actions and had enough perspective to see the humor in a friend's December–May marriage.

> A dear friend of mine who was separated and subsequently divorced fell in love with a woman considerably his junior. He's my age, 52 to 54, and she's in her 20s. Their wedding was the funniest thing you've ever seen. I was best man and the wedding party was made up of these old guys all paired up with young lovelies. As we walked down the aisle, it was like six young ladies getting married to their dads. It was really funny. I mean bald, gray-haired guys with paunches arm in arm with these blond, tight little lovelies.
>
> I'm not a psychologist, but this clearly has to do with how men feel about their age and attractiveness as they get older—a younger person who's attracted to you makes you feel less old. I experienced that during my separation when I had a couple of dates with women maybe fifteen years younger than me. It was nice, it was neat, it was fun. But I didn't think of it as a permanent kind of thing because the difference in our development was a direct re-

flection of our age difference. But it felt good. And there's no question that a young lovely lady on your arm is an arm charm.

Married father, 52

The real irony of midlife change is there is often a reintegration of masculine and feminine traits. Events associated with menopause and turning 50 can make a woman more assertive and independent, while her male counterpart may react to his life changes by becoming more sensitive and nurturing.

It's frustrating to watch my wife go through menopause and not be able to do anything to help. I'd like her to feel as well as I do when I get up every morning. When I go to bed at night, I'm confident that I'll feel great the next day. But my wife just doesn't have that same sense of security, and it makes it tough for her on a day-to-day basis. I feel sorry for her not being able to control what's happening to her body.

Married father, 56

Timing is never perfect, but it is reassuring to know that men do soften a little with age.

What? Male Menopause?

In truth, there is no such thing as male menopause. Because men do not menstruate, the term is ridiculous when it comes to describing male physical changes at midlife. Nevertheless, as they age, men do experience a drop in hormones—both testosterone and growth hormones. The major difference between women's and men's midlife transition is the rate at which their respective hormone production declines. For women, the drop-off is relatively precipitous, even without surgery. The two- to ten-year time span for perimenopause is quicker than you think. Men, however, experience a more gradual hormonal decline over a thirty- to forty-year period.

Now that women are becoming more vocal about menopause and the effects of aging that go along with it, men are taking a furtive look at what might be in store for them. Most men are unaware of their scientifically proven hormonal decline. Not much has appeared in the press to date, and with their manhood closely aligned to physical prowess, men are not likely to stir up this issue. Like this man who admits to some change, most men will cope with the truly aggravating aspects of body changes and ignore the rest.

I've noticed different things, funny things. The slowdown by a step—you're playing tennis and you see the ball and your body doesn't even move—it's a step behind. And the computer printout in your brain doesn't work quite as well when you're trying to remember some things. I also sleep differently and notice I'm a little more tired when I'm doing physical stuff. But the real annoyance is interruptions during the night. If anyone ever invents a way to avoid getting up to pee during the night, it would be terrific.
Married father, 54

Hormonal decline is real, and in Europe, for example, the concept of a male climacteric is well accepted. It is so well accepted that it is called *andropause,* after the class of androgen hormones that includes testosterone. Researchers in the United States are just beginning to take male hormone decline seriously and are toying with names like *testopause* or *somatopause—somato* is the scientific prefix for growth hormone—to describe male midlife change.

No matter what you call it, male hormonal decline is not insignificant. For instance, testosterone is the primary male hormone responsible for hair growth, libido, sexual performance, bone growth, and muscle development. Its counterpart, growth hormone, plays a key role in a man's ability to burn off sugar and fat. Take away some of these powerful hormones, even at a slow rate, and there is bound to be a noticeable effect.

Of course there are a lot of physical changes. You lose your hair and your back hurts a little bit. But I work out and manage to stay in pretty good shape. I used to be a big jogger and now my knees are gone—I can't do that, so you do something else. Every once in a while I pass a mirror or a window and think, What's happening—my father's here, what's he . . . *Then I realize,* Hey, wait a minute—that's me.

Married father, 56

In a well-researched article in the July 1992 issue of M *Magazine* titled "Do Men Go Through Menopause?" author Randi Hutter Epstein, M.D., reported, "Testosterone levels can begin to creep downward at age 40, but by and large, testosterone and growth hormone don't start waning significantly until around age 60—some ten years after female menopause." Other recent studies suggest that testosterone can decline by as much as 30 to 40 percent between the ages of 48 and 70 and that one-third of men between the ages of 60 and 70 are deficient in growth hormone.

Too bad this long-term decline does not bring on a hot flash or two. Instead, men with lower testosterone levels may have a broad range of symptoms, including a decline in muscle mass and strength, a buildup of body fat, the loss of bone density, flagging energy, lowered fertility, and fading virility. (See Chapter 7, "Sex," for more specific effects on sexual performance.) Further, according to Dr. Jeffrey Jackson at the University of Texas, Southwestern, in Dallas, men with low levels of testosterone are 6.5 times more likely than those with normal levels to suffer hip fractures. Midlife paunches and flabbier biceps and quads may also be attributable to decreased growth hormone. Then there is the emotional side of the picture. Some recent, but very modest, research suggests a connection between testosterone and mood. It seems that testosterone can affect a man's outlook on life, energy level, assertiveness, powers of concentration, and his overall sense of well-being.

Amazingly, for as little research that has been done on menopause, even less exists on andropause. Many of the scientific conclusions are based on small studies, some of which are only with animals. Dr. Epstein gives an excellent example of the current research situation: "There are some studies on animals, and a limited number on humans, that suggest a link between *extreme* losses of testosterone and decreases in muscle strength, muscle mass, bone formation, appetite, sex drive, and facial hair. However, these results, in both mice and men, were found in the presence of drastic decreases in testosterone—the kind of loss linked with chronic illness. It's not clear whether the information can be extrapolated to the typical older man who falls somewhere in between the hearty 25-year-old and the sick 90-year-old on the testosterone scale. Nor is it clear how much the most virile mouse has in common with a man."

As you can see, male hormone decline is a new and potentially lucrative issue. There are rumors of hormone replacement therapy for men, and study proposals are being submitted to the National Institutes for Health on a regular basis. Men will have to face similar issues to women in terms of hormone replacement therapy. The side effects of taking testosterone include an increased risk of certain kinds of cancer, particularly prostate cancer. Evidence also exists that hormones may actually thicken the blood, thus increasing the risk of heart disease. The question of male hormone replacement therapy will be up in the air for a long time, and it will be fascinating to see how men deal with the ongoing uncertainty.

How to Talk to Men About Menopause

After reading the earlier part of this chapter, you are well aware that a man is not interested in chapter and verse on menopause. Yet, he might be curious about menopausal issues that land close to home and affect his daily life and relationship with you. According to the statistics, he really does care. So, the conundrum is to figure out his interest and get the right kind of information across to him.

Having successfully interviewed many women for this book, I was surprised to find that I needed to completely alter my technique when talking to men. Whereas women were anxious to answer almost any kind of question, men were at their best when responding to issues that affected them directly. Furthermore, men had a shorter attention span and were less likely to speculate on a subject they were uncertain about. This may seem strikingly obvious, but it was harder than you might imagine to determine exactly what men care about and how to get through to them, especially when it comes to women and menopause.

Take the Male Viewpoint

If you can put yourself in men's shoes for a few minutes, you will find that only a small number of menopausal factors have a direct bearing on their lives, namely,

- Sex.
- Hot flashes.
- Mood swings.
- Loss of reproductive ability.

Focus on these issues and you will have a good chance of striking a receptive nerve or two.

Take sex, for example. More than likely, a man's concern about your vaginal dryness will be limited to how it impacts your sex life. Yes, he really does care that sex might hurt you, but he is also far more interested in solving the problem than dwelling on the physical aspects of why it is happening. The same can be said for excessive bleeding that might curtail your sex life or even a temporary loss of libido. As mentioned in Chapter 7, "Sex," it is important to be clear about why sex may not be on the top of your list at the moment. This father of two gives a good description of what it might be like to be left in the dark.

> I've heard of women using menopause as an excuse not to have sex with their husbands anymore, maybe because they have had a lousy relationship for years. All of a sudden a woman turns to her husband and says, "Forget about it, Harry—don't bother me anymore. I'm in menopause." I imagine that could be very troubling to a man because now you're dealing with an issue that affects him as well. He probably doesn't understand menopause, maybe he's confused, maybe he doesn't know what to do. He

thinks he's being rejected, he thinks his wife is sick—there are all kinds of things that can build up in your mind if you don't know what's really going on.

Married father, 57

You must also try to think about hot flashes from a man's perspective if you want to get the support you need. Does he truly care that you constantly change clothes to keep from looking like you just walked in off the Sahara Desert? Will he share your embarrassment over sweating in public? Probably not. However, you can bet that if you share a bed and suffer from repeated night sweats, he will be sympathetic to your feelings of sleep deprivation. Unfortunately he may be just as cranky as you, but he at least will understand firsthand some of what you are experiencing.

Mood swings are another matter. If you are able to identify "a bad day" or reply with an angry response that was out of character and give warning that episodes like these may be more frequent in the future, you will probably get a man's attention. He is definitely affected by different and undesirable behavior on your part and would probably be relieved to understand why it is happening. The key is to try to disassociate unusual moodiness from your normal disposition, tag it, and offer it up as evidence of a menopausal transition. It is still part of who you are, but by holding it up to separate scrutiny by you and your mate, you may get more support and understanding if you emphasize the temporary nature of this phenomenon.

For some women, no longer being able to have children is a big plus, with positive implications for contraception and less complicated sexual activity. For others, it is a major crisis either in terms of identity or loss of the chance to become pregnant. Either way, your mate will be affected to some degree. In discussions, try to focus on the aspects that will have a direct bearing on him. You are the one who is going through menopause, yet your ability to frame up the implications in a husband-oriented fashion will determine the amount of your mate's empathy.

Be the Aggressor

Talking about menopause to a man is one time when a woman is definitely in charge of the situation. No matter how sensitive and caring he may seem, no man is about to step into uncharted waters and initiate a conversation about menopause. With his lack of knowledge, a man is not likely to deliberately put himself at a disadvantage in a one-on-one conversation with a woman.

This means you will have to take the first step and the second and third one as well. You hold all the cards—knowledge of the subject, how it may affect a man, and what to do about it—even if you are uncertain about your exact course of action.

Once you have focused on what menopausal issue you want to discuss with a man, you then need to turn it into a highway billboard. You know, the kind you can read, understand, and respond to within ten seconds while you are driving 60 miles an hour. This is not a joke. By now you certainly know firsthand how little a man wants to know about the details and emotions most women find to be at the center of their thoughts. Do not make a hard task more difficult. Men are smart and can grasp complex concepts if you take the time to properly present them in an unmuddled way. Pick your shots carefully and then deliver them in a direct and concise fashion. If this is done right, your mate will be all ears.

A little help from a disinterested third party can also go a long way to furthering communication. Short magazine articles or several highlighted pages from a book with your notes in the margin can provide a man with enormous insight. It also allows him to learn about what is important to you in a very nonthreatening way. With this passive mode of pass-along information, a man avoids feeling like he knows nothing at all about women and menopause.

Set Yourself Up for Success

You are the best judge of what bothers you most and with heightened awareness probably understand the impact it has on those around you. However, before you open any discussion on the topic, try to figure out what, if anything, your mate can do to help. If it is something that only you can solve and really does not involve or affect a man directly, you are better off choosing a different issue—one that he can do something about. After all, the last thing a man needs is to hear about a problem and feel powerless to help.

Once you have zeroed in on an appropriate menopausal issue, present it in a way that lets your mate know what is expected of him in terms of response. Be specific and spell it out. For example, if you are discussing sex and your difficulty with vaginal dryness, let him know that an additional ten minutes of foreplay will make all the difference in the world.

Last, and perhaps most important, is how you respond to his effort to help. No matter that it was not exactly what you had in mind, it was an attempt to be supportive and helpful. It is essential that you reinforce this positive behavior if you expect to have it happen again. Instead of focusing on how your mate should have responded, give him credit for making the effort. Fine-tuning can come later, after your husband has had a chance to feel good about his action.

As a final suggestion, photocopy a section of this book written exclusively for men and give it to your mate, your date, your business associate, or your friend to read. "Seven Points Every Man Should Know About Menopause" can be found in Appendix 1. By reading these few pages, a man will be able to get a quick understanding of menopause and the issues that are important to women. Encourage the men in your life to read it.

Chapter Ten

How to Get Good Treatment

As simple as it may sound, finding a doctor in whom you have confidence as well as feel comfortable and have a rapport with is one of the most difficult tasks for many women at midlife. With all the changes happening to your body, it may seem unclear just what kind of medical care is appropriate. Furthermore, as midlife patients, women have a greater level of self-confidence and are more demanding about the quality of care they receive. Add to that the wide spectrum of physicians' attitudes about menopause that can turn a routine doctor's appointment into a half hour of uncertainty and frustration and you have a real problem. Consequently, many menopausal women find themselves dissatisfied with their current level of medical care and go from doctor to doctor in quest of the medical advice and counsel they need.

To solve this problem without spending a fortune on doctor's bills will take some effort on your part. More and more women have discovered that they must take a stronger role in the management of their medical care. Those who do usually end up with a group of medical professionals who can be relied on for sound advice, good health care, and solid emotional support.

Choosing and Working with a Practitioner

Many of us grew up under the care of a family doctor, usually a comforting sort who knew our parents and siblings. In addition to conducting examinations and prescribing medication, the family doctor often had an extended role—dispensing advice on subjects from getting through puberty to how to get along with friends at school.

The heyday of the general practitioner is long gone, and it has been supplanted by the era of the specialist, a physician devoted to one particular area of medicine, and with good reason. Medicine has advanced to a more complex and sophisticated stage than ever before.

Patients have changed, too. As a group, they no longer view doctors as godlike individuals not to be challenged. Instead they ask a lot of questions, read articles and books to get more information, and tune in to television specials on specific diseases, medical insurance, malpractice, and the latest medical breakthroughs.

It is not surprising that many women in their early 40s have already met with confusion and frustration in finding the right practitioner for their changing medical needs. They go from one doctor to another and often emerge dissatisfied—not because the medical community has become incompetent overnight. More likely these situations are a result of poor rapport, inadequate communication, or choosing the wrong specialist.

In studies of doctor–patient relationships, 90 percent of the patient complaints revolve around poor communication and the doctor's

- Lack of compassion.
- Infrequent eye contact.

- Humiliation of the patient.
- Use of confusing medical jargon.

To add insult to injury, studies find that physicians tend to interrupt patients constantly and not give them an opportunity to explain what is really bothering them.

In many instances, women who have had a smooth relationship with a doctor suddenly find themselves in a real mess once they bring up a problem that requires more than a blood test and a prescription. Unfortunately, this woman's experience is not unusual.

> *I had a blood test before I went on vacation because I was really upset with what was happening with my period and the pain and soreness in my breasts that seemed to go along with it. I just felt something was wrong. After I got back, I checked back in with my doctor. I walked into the office and said, "I haven't had my period in two months. Am I pregnant?" She said, "Pregnant? Looking at your blood tests, you're menopausal. You have no estrogen left in your body and you're probably going to be finished menstruating for good in a few months." At which point, she tossed some hormone replacement pills my way along with a pamphlet. And that was it.*
>
> Married mother, 46

Given their collective knowledge, a different kind of relationship needs to be established between doctor and patient, a relationship that is more open and up-to-date. First, you have to fully understand your expectations in consulting a medical professional. The next step is to find the right kind of doctor for your needs.

What to Expect from Your Practitioner
When you spend time and money to consult a specialist for professional advice, you expect clear, understandable results and a basic level of service. This holds true whether it is a contractor

to redo the kitchen, a financial planner to examine money management, or a tennis instructor to improve your game. At the minimum, you will probably get what you contracted for. You might luck out and get all of that plus good service, attention to your needs, and a friendly attitude thrown in for good measure. However, if the results are not up to your expectations, you will probably make your feelings known and do everything in your power to get what you paid for.

Consulting a medical practitioner is no different. You "hire" a practitioner for professional advice, treatment, and counsel. You should not be satisfied until you get just that. Yet many of us become sheepish the minute we walk into a doctor's office.

Here are some suggestions for getting the most out of your doctor–patient relationship:

- *Help your doctor hear your needs and understand your problem.* There is nothing worse than a doctor who treats you impersonally, as if you were just another statistic. Yes, your situation is probably not new or unique in terms of the medical community, but it is new and different for you. A practitioner should take the time to really listen, without interruption, in order to understand your problem and how it is affecting you. Physicians are notorious for interrupting patients.

  Most patients make matters worse by not presenting their physical complaints in order of magnitude. Often, the thing that bothers you the most is held back and saved for the grand finale. With constant interruption, you may not even get to the third act. Sometimes, you might actually have to take charge of the conversation in order to make yourself heard. This means you need to overcome any feelings of embarrassment, anxiety, and timidity. There is no question you will end up with better medical care if your real problems are heard and understood. Make sure you have a doctor who listens more and talks less. Remember, this is what you are paying for.

- *Insist on explanations in plain English.* Getting a response from a doctor in terms that you can understand is often a real challenge. Because medical explanations are usually given in technical terms, you can easily feel stupid about not understanding what they mean. Stop right here. There is nothing wrong with your brain. Insist on a clear explanation of tests and procedures necessary for diagnosis, including a description of what you can expect in terms of immediate and long-term discomfort. Do not buy into something you cannot understand.
- *Press for direct and honest answers to your questions.* Would you let a contractor working on your kitchen get away with giving you half-baked answers to your questions? What about a subordinate at work? Do not let it happen in the doctor's office either. Make sure the response you get answers the question you ask. If not, ask again until you get the answer.

  You can also help in this process by creating a list of questions beforehand. Review your previous medical visit in your mind and focus on which medical decisions need to be considered for this visit. Then write your questions down and do not feel stupid about carrying them with you to your appointment.

  Frustrated in her efforts to be heard after visiting several doctors, this woman gives the following advice:

You talk to your doctor and say, "Look, I'm in my 40s now and I'm going to go through menopause . . . What's going to happen to me? What kinds of physical changes should I be aware of? What are my chances, given my family history, of getting heart disease, of developing cancer? Are my bones going to thin? Should I take calcium? How do I find out where I am on the scale? Am I a candidate for osteoporosis?" Asking questions isn't going to put a hex on you. For your $75–150, you're entitled to some questions and some answers. And then it's not just take that Pap smear and leave. Everyone has a Pap smear and then waits for the notice in *the mail or the phone call. If you detect cells that are abnormal, what do you do? I mean nobody knows. Because nobody ever asks the question. You just lie on the table and let them do it and focus on hoping that it doesn't hurt. When you go once a year, talk to your doctor and express some of your concerns.*

Single woman, 42

Insist on an opportunity to ask your questions when you are sitting down in the office, fully clothed, and have a reasonable allotment of time. If you need to, write the doctor's answers down as well. In that way you can be sure you get the information you need.

• *Find a doctor with a friendly and approachable attitude.* Although it is unlikely that your doctor will become your best friend, there is no reason to put up with an indifferent, hostile, or arrogant demeanor. Dealing with physical problems is not fun and often evokes feelings of fear and insecurity. This is a time when you want to feel as though someone cares. Research has shown that empathetic doctors are more satisfied with their work, are less likely to be sued for malpractice, and have patients who are happier with their medical care. Keep looking until you find a doctor who cares about you.

After my doctor had explained the alternatives, I still felt dissatisfied and frustrated. I didn't like any of them. Yet I knew that he had told me about everything that was available. "How would you like it if you were a woman?" I asked. He said, "You're probably right, but I don't like going bald very much either."

Single woman, 49

How to Find a Practitioner for Midlife Care

When it comes to seeking medical help, it is usually obvious what kind of doctor to consult: for a sore back you go to an orthopedist; for a toothache, the dentist. But what about menopause? Who do you go to for professional advice? A gynecologist?

An internist? A gerontologist? A cardiologist? An orthopedist? What kind of medical care do you look for?

Being menopausal can put you in an odd situation. After all, you are not suffering from a disease. You may not even have any signs of menopause. Yet, now that you know some of the health issues associated with menopause, you surely want to get the best medical advice you can find. Even with all the new interest in menopause, it is unlikely that you will find a listing of specialists in the yellow pages. As a specific branch of medicine, midlife or menopausal care has still not made the list.

Perhaps a new approach is in order. Instead of looking to your gynecologist for your primary medical care, you may want to consider consulting an internist for your nongynecological needs. As you approach menopause, you will discover a shift in your medical focus from issues related to your reproductive system to other facets of your body. Internists are qualified to handle a wide variety of medical complaints, including rudimentary gynecological care. In fact, most women over 55 see an internist as their primary physician and consult more specialized doctors as needed. Ideally, you will be able to find a physician with a holistic approach to your medical care—one who evaluates your medical complaint as just one factor in how you function both physically and emotionally.

Because it may be difficult to find a "menopause specialist," here are some guidelines to help you select a doctor for your midlife needs:

- *Determine the doctor's attitude toward menopause.* Set up an appointment to discuss the subject of menopause in general. Without discussing your specific symptoms, you should be able to get an indication of the doctor's feelings about hot flashes, aging, prescribed treatment, and overall viewpoint on menopause. If the doctor refers to menopause as a disease or says you are too young to be going through menopause, you are probably not going to be happy with an ongoing relationship.

- *Check the average age of patients.* This is an easy and quick indicator of the kind of practice a doctor has. What percentage are women 40 to 60 years old?
- *Understand any biases or predisposition toward treatment.* This may elicit a defensive response from the potential doctor, but it is useful to know the following:
  - Does this doctor prescribe hormone replacement therapy for the majority of patients?
  - What is the doctor's feeling about alternative forms of treatment?
  - How often are hysterectomies performed?
  - What is the doctor's attitude toward retaining ovaries?
  - Are biopsies a routine practice?

  These are all routine questions that you should feel comfortable asking in an initial interview. If the doctor is noncommittal on issues or not forthcoming with answers, it is a good indicator that you will not receive all the information you need about your own medical care.
- *Investigate the doctor's training and areas of specialization.* This may be a little more difficult to do, and you may get a better response by talking to the nurses in the office about the following:
  - How much experience has this doctor had with menopausal women?
  - How up-to-date is the doctor on the latest issues relating to midlife health care: hormone replacement therapy, osteoporosis, heart disease, exercise, and nutrition?
  - What percentage of the practice is dedicated to menopausal women?
  - What associations and special medical interest groups does the doctor belong to?

Menopause Clinics

Because of the large number of women reaching menopause in the next twenty years, the medical community is paying special attention to the health needs of midlife women. There is a sharp increase in menopause research, new studies on osteoporosis, and more investigation of women and heart disease. To keep pace with this trend, clinics with specialties in health care related to menopause have started to appear throughout the country.

Unfortunately, not all clinics are created equal, and although many offer appropriate health services to midlife women, some are merely hastily put together and do not offer comprehensive menopausal care. Currently, there is no standard for services a menopause clinic should provide. Consequently, care ranges from a single doctor who refers patients for additional services to a multidisciplinary consortium of professionals who handle physical, social, and emotional problems. The following sample of menopause clinics will give you an idea of what you can expect when seeking out this kind of specialized health care.

Hormone Clinic/Mature Women's Clinic
Albert Einstein College of Medicine
1300 Morris Park Avenue
Bronx, NY 10461
(718) 430-3152
Ruth Freeman, M.D.

Services Offered: Full diagnostic testing, including blood hormone levels, bone densitometry, mammography, nutritional and psychological counseling, and social services. Several gynecologic and medical endocrinologists on staff are trained in prescribing and monitoring hormone replacement therapy (HRT).

Average Age of Patients: Patients range in age from 19 to 79 years old. The clinic specializes in premature ovarian failure (and has an ovum donor program) as well as in treating menopause and postmenopausal osteoporosis.

Concerns of Menopausal Patients: Hot flashes, vaginal dryness, and concerns about the effects of menopause on the bones.

Follow-Up Services Offered: All necessary follow-up of patients on HRT is done. In the first year, patients on HRT are seen every three months to adjust the dosage. Thereafter, these patients are seen every six months.

Support Group Services: Patients, many of whom come from far away, are sent to outside support groups. The clinic is moving to a larger facility, however, and will soon have in-house classes and support sessions for patients.

> Cleveland Menopause Clinic
> 5850 Landerbrook Drive
> Mayfield Heights, OH 44124
> (216) 442-4747
> Wulf Utian, M.D.

Services Offered: Comprehensive menopause program, offering a full spectrum of women's health care. Services include screening, bone densitometry, mammography, ultrasonography. The multidisciplinary staff offers a full range of therapies, including HRT and alternatives.

Average Age of Patients: All age ranges (premature and normal menopause).

Concerns of Menopausal Patients: Hot flashes and vaginal atrophy.

Follow-Up Services Offered: An individualized follow-up is based on a sixteen-page questionnaire and medical evaluation. Patients are seen regularly for preventive care (e.g., if they are at high risk for osteoporosis, breast cancer, or ovarian cancer) and to monitor therapies.

Support Group Services: The clinic conducts a traveling menopause education program.

The Menopause Clinic
University of California, San Diego
3969 4th Avenue
San Diego, CA 92103
(619) 453-3210 ("hot flash" line)
Sonia Hamburger, B.A., coordinator

Services Offered: A ten-year-old menopause educational and so-
cial/psychological support service offered through the department
of reproductive endocrinology. Up-to-the-minute information
on HRT, sexuality, breast self-examination and mammography,
surgery, and osteoporosis is disseminated. The clinic holds four-
hour group sessions for menopausal women every two weeks;
groups are limited to five women. Sessions consist of education
(including talks by an R.N./Ph.D. and a doctor), the sharing of
experiences, and advice on how to deal with doctors. Women
are encouraged to return to their own doctors for further evaluation and treatment. Referrals can be made if requested.

Average Age of Patients: 40s to 50s; most are perimenopausal.

Follow-Up Services Offered: Women come to the group session
only once; after that they can call the "hot flash" line if they
have questions.

Women to Women
1 Pleasant Street
Yarmouth, ME 04096
(207) 846-6163
Christiane Northrup, M.D.

Services Offered: A full-service gynecology practice with six pro-
viders. One nurse/practitioner specializes in treating perimenopausal women. Other specialties include PMS, endometriosis,
breast cancer, and colposcopy (examination of the vagina and
cervix using an instrument with a magnifying lens inserted into
the vagina) for abnormal Pap smears. The clinic emphasizes a

holistic approach to treatment—for example, natural progesterone cream as an alternative to HRT—and the patient as keeper of her own health care. Menopausal women are offered standard procedures such as blood tests and arm span measurements. Referrals are made for bone densitometry, mammography, and lab services.

Average Age of Patients: All ages.

Concerns of Menopausal Patients: Hot flashes, irregular bleeding, and mood swings.

Follow-Up Services Offered: Long-term.

Support Group Services: Periodic educational workshops are offered on menopause, nutrition, and creating good health, with time for group discussions. The clinic has developed the "Creating Health Guide" and audiocassettes on menopause, endometriosis, and PMS.

Penny Wise Budoff, M.D.
Women's Health Services
Affiliated with North Shore University Hospital
4300 Hempstead Turnpike
Bethpage, NY 11714
(516) 579-6900

Services Offered: A full-service women's health center; multispecialty care. Tests offered to menopausal women include mammography, bone densitometry, X rays, blood tests, and cancer screening. The clinic offers HRT and alternatives, such as calcitonin and bisphosphonates. Two osteoporosis research studies are currently under way; if accepted into the protocol, patients receive free care.

Average Age of Patients: All ages.

Concerns of Menopausal Patients: Hot flashes, vaginal dryness, night sweats, osteoporosis, and cardiovascular disease.

Follow-Up Services Offered: All patients over 40 years of age are seen every six months. Both in-depth medical and gynecological care are offered.

Support Group Services: Dr. Budoff lectures at North Shore University Hospital as well as at her center. Patients are referred to community support groups.

> Women's Hospital
> University of Southern California Women's Health Center
> 1240 North Mission Road
> Los Angeles, CA 90033
> (213) 222-4028
> Rogerio Lobo, M.D.

Services Offered: This menopause "clinic" is only involved in conducting studies of unapproved pharmacological agents on menopausal women. No routine care is offered. Depending on research study protocol, mammograms, blood tests, physical examinations, HRT, and so on may be offered.

Average Age of Patients: Healthy women from 52 to 60 years of age, some in their 40s. Patients receive free care upon acceptance to a study.

Concerns of Menopausal Patients: Hot flashes, depression, mood swings, fatigue, and a fear of osteoporosis.

Follow-Up Services Offered: The follow-up depends on study protocol.

Support Group Services: None.

In addition to generalized menopause clinics, specialty clinics, such as the following, that focus on osteoporosis are starting to become popular. There is an enormous advantage to using the services of a specialty clinic because you will usually get the best care available for a specific need, performed by professionals dedicated only to that specialty. Furthermore, because practitioners working in specialized clinics see patients with similar problems, their expertise is usually more finely tuned.

Osteoporosis Prevention Center
University of Connecticut Health Center
Farm Hollow
Farmington, CT 06030
(203) 679-3850
Lawrence Raisz, M.D.

Services Offered: A multidisciplinary team approach to osteoporosis, both to clinical disease and prevention. The center offers bone densitometry, blood tests, calcium workup, exercise programs, drug therapy, and counseling. Research is also conducted —prevention and clinical therapy trials, plus biochemistry behind osteoporosis investigations.

There are two basic programs:

1. *Osteoporosis Prevention Program.* This program evaluates healthy women for osteoporosis risk. First visit: set up testing; second visit: review test results, develop prevention program. The majority of patients are postmenopausal women.
2. *Osteoporosis Clinic.* This program is for patients who are at high risk for osteoporosis, already have osteoporosis, or have fractures. These patients receive full testing, evaluation, and follow-up.

Average Age of Patients: Women and men of all ages.

Concerns of Menopausal Patients: The fear of osteoporosis, back pain. Most women come to the clinic to find help in their decision making concerning HRT.

Follow-Up Services Offered: Patients receive individualized follow-up. For postmenopausal women, follow-up depends on whether they are at risk for osteoporosis. If they are taking HRT, they are followed annually. If no bone loss is evident, they are followed every two to three years; if bone loss is evident, annual visits are recommended.

Support Group Services: If necessary, patients can be referred to in-house mental health services.

Osteoporosis Center
Hospital for Special Surgery
535 East 70th Street
New York, NY 10021
(212) 606-1588
Theresa Galsworthy, R.N., O.N.C.

Services Offered: A comprehensive bone evaluation by a team of doctors, including bone densitometry testing of the hip, spine, and forearm; spinal X rays; blood tests; and bone biopsies. First visit: set up testing; second visit: a one-hour review of test results, and development of an individualized program. The clinic offers counseling on menopause issues such as HRT, osteoporosis prevention, nutrition, and exercise. The clinic conducts osteoporosis research.

Average Age of Patients: Women and men between 40 and 60.

Concerns of Menopausal Patients: Mostly asymptomatic; some may have back pain. Most women come to the clinic to find help in their decision making concerning HRT.

Follow-Up Services Offered: A high percentage of revisits are to track menopausal women for bone loss.

Support Group Services: The clinic plans to start a support group for menopause and osteoporosis.

Center for Bone Diseases
Duke University Medical Center
Box 3470
Durham, NC 27710
(800) 831-8006, (919) 286-4476
Kristine Harper, M.D.

Services Offered: An endocrine clinic, staffed by endocrinologists who see patients with all bone disorders. The primary diagnosis is osteoporosis. The clinic offers bone densitometry, X rays, bone biopsies, HRT, and alternative treatments. The clinic also serves as a research center.

In addition to testing, evaluation, and diagnosis, the clinic offers a four-day outpatient osteoporosis program (out-of-town patients stay near the medical center) limited to three to five patients per group. On the first day, patients receive intensive evaluation by the full staff—physician, physical therapist, social worker, nutritionist, and nurses. The second, third, and fourth days are devoted to patient education and individualized exercise programs.

Average Age of Patients: Women and men of all ages.

Concerns of Menopausal Patients: Because this is a tertiary medical center, many patients come because they have already suffered fractures, have osteoporosis symptoms, or are frail. A few come for prevention purposes.

Follow-Up Services Offered: If the patient goes in for diagnosis and testing, follow-up is individualized. If patients sign up for the four-day program, they are followed at three months, seven and one-half months, and one year, then semiannually or annually after that. Because this is a specialty clinic, patients return to their primary physicians for regular care.

Support Group Services: There are no ongoing support group services. The social worker can refer patients to community groups.

For those who are interested in a total immersion program, there are retreats dedicated to the subject of menopause and its specific impact on your body. One is an offshoot of a spa program, and the other is a combination physical, emotional, and spiritual sojourn focusing on midlife issues. Undoubtedly, more programs like these will appear in the next few years, and they can be quite helpful if you have the time and money to try one.

Midlife Women's Health
  Program
Canyon Ranch Tucson
8600 East Rockcliff Road
Tucson, AZ 85715
(602) 749-9655
Elizabeth Lee Vliet, M.D.

Canyon Ranch
91 Kemble Street
Lenox, MA 02140
(413) 637-4100
Tildabeth Doscher, M.D.

Services Offered: In addition to a 90-minute seminar on women's health issues and menopause, the program offers a preventive health medical evaluation. Depending on your health, it can include a complete physical, metabolic profile (thyroid function, blood count, lipid profile, and resting metabolic rate to determine appropriate daily caloric intake), cardiac stress test, hormonal evaluation (endocrine status), bone densitometry, mammogram, and other appropriate evaluations. A board-certified endocrinologist/gynecologist is available for consultation as needed. Individual consultations with a registered dietitian and exercise physiologist are available to develop nutrition and fitness programs.

After testing, women are given their current health status and recommendations for reducing disease risk. The program emphasizes preventive medicine.

Average Age of Attendees: 35 to 50 years (perimenopausal women); 50 to 75 years (menopausal women).

Concerns of Menopausal Attendees: Mood changes, memory loss, weight gain, vaginal discomfort, and hot flashes. Women complain that their physicians do not listen to them. Many of the perimenopausal women complain about worsening PMS and an increased number of migraines. Many also request bone densitometry.

Follow-Up Services Offered: A written summary of medical evaluation and recommendations is given as well as ongoing encouragement to help the patient take charge of her medical care, including instructions for interviewing physicians and specialists.

Copper Feather Institute for Midlife Enhancement
1200 North Beaver Street
Flagstaff, AZ 86001
(602) 773-2559
Lana L. Holstein, M.D.

Services Offered: Held in a quiet resort facility, this is a three-day retreat focusing on midlife issues involving the mind, body, and spirit. The goal of the retreat is to put all of these issues together in order to have a larger picture and gain perspective on what is happening at midlife. Groups are limited to thirty people. Participants undergo a blood drawing for cholesterol and lipid profiles, thyroid profile, kidney and liver studies, and hormonal analysis; no other physical tests are given. Data are also collected on your lifework and special interests. The focus is on education, didactic and experiential exercises, discussions on osteoporosis, heart disease, menopausal indicators, and so on.

Average Age of Attendees: Women in their late 40s and early 50s; the range is 30 to 78 years old.

Concerns of Menopausal Attendees: Sexuality at midlife and the loss of sex drive.

Follow-Up Services Offered: This is a one-time retreat; however, the institute sends alumni information once a year. An alumni retreat is also offered and serves as a second-level course on midlife issues.

Elizabeth Paul Center
8600 East Rockcliff Drive
Tucson, AZ 85715
(602) 749-5757
Elizabeth Lee Vliet, M.D., medical director

Different from any of the clinics or programs mentioned above, a new concept in women's midlife health care, the Elizabeth Paul Center, appeared on the scene in May 1993. Based in Tucson, Arizona, and developed by women professionals, the Elizabeth Paul Center is dedicated to patients as partners in health care, and advocates a totally integrated approach to achieving this goal. This means that patients have the opportunity to become educated about menopause and other physical, psychological, and spiritual midlife issues, while at the same time they can take advantage of courses of treatment from comprehensive "whole person assessment" to individualized health plans, including nutrition and exercise programs, hormone replacement therapy, acupuncture, and meditation. Because the Elizabeth Paul Center does not advocate a singular approach to treatment, patients are truly treated as individuals in all facets of their health care. Hopefully, the center is a prototype of future clinics in that it offers:

- Full inpatient/outpatient clinical services.
- An information clearinghouse for women's midlife issues, with library facilities and networking opportunities.
- An educational facility for ongoing continuing-education courses for health professionals in all fields.
- Clinical research programs.
- A referral service with information about locally available resources and services for women unable to travel to Arizona.
- Outreach educational seminars for communities across the country.
- Videotapes, audiotapes, and books on women's health topics, reviewed for accuracy and up-to-date information.

Professional Organizations

If all else fails and you cannot get any satisfaction from current doctors, recommendations from friends, or various clinics and hospital services, you can try contacting professional organizations. In addition to the North American Menopause Society and the American College of Obstetrics and Gynecology, you might also get creative and contact various menopause or health-related newsletters for names of doctors (see Appendix 2, "Resources"). All of this requires serious amounts of time and energy on your part, but there is no question that your long-term health is worth the effort.

Chapter Eleven

Middle Age and the Next Thirty Years

Of course we do not expect to find any virus-disease from without as peculiar to the change of Life. The English name—change of life—is singularly appropriate: It is what its name implies and nothing more. The woman who is really in sound health—i.e., of good constitution—is quite as well at and after the change as before. A good constitution does not then become bad.
—J. Compton Burnett, M.D.,
The Change of Life in Women, 1898

Going through menopause is like hitting the big time. All of a sudden you feel like you are in the major leagues. You are finally an adult and no one mistakes you for an overgrown 20-year-old. Although you may not be able to see the light at the end of the tunnel, you certainly know that it is there. By middle age, you and the world know who you are—your previous accomplishments, friendships, family relationships, all speak for you.

Now that you have arrived, you may find yourself in a strange state of limbo wondering just where you are: "If this is middle age, how do I fit in?" The confusion felt by this woman is common.

I've always thought that middle-aged people are very stable—they usually have a 9 to 5 job and are settled in their lives. They're solid, they're adult, and they also gain weight and don't look great anymore. But I'm middle-aged and don't fit that picture at all. I look younger and am still pretty effervescent. It's like I haven't arrived, almost like I've failed in some way, and it's very confusing.

Single mother, 49

Pictures of Women at Middle Age

Face it: Our great-grandmothers, grandmothers, and mothers all went through middle age, but at a different time, in a different place in the world. Today, middle age is a time of life that probably needs some redefinition. Was your mother behaving the way you do when she was your age? Did she still play tennis in her 50s or go out for a 3-mile run in her 40s? How conscious was she of what she ate? Did she even know about fat grams? And sex? Were she and your father still getting it on after 50? Did she actively seek out men after your father was no longer around? What about work? Did she have a career and continue it until retirement in her 60s or start a second career in her 50s?

Rock and roll. These are the no-nonsense '90s, and women in their 40s, 50s, and 60s are a new breed. Remember how appalling it was to think of turning 40? Well, here you are and then some. Aside from some physical and emotional blips associated with the aging process, all in all, middle age is not so bad and certainly not an impediment to getting on with your life in fine style.

For some reason, however, society's view of aging women has not changed with the times. The subject here may be middle age, but attitudes about women and aging stem from the Middle or Dark Ages. Since what seems like the beginning of time, aging women have been viewed negatively. Yes, there are some positive images of older women: the earth mother, goddesses of spring and summer, the personification of the wholeness of life. More often, however middle-aged women take it on the chin. According to Dr. Rita Ransohoff in her book *Venus After Forty* (Far Hills, NJ: New Horizon Press, 1987), "Woman, in her loss of fertility, is equated with aging and dying."

Negative myths about older women abound in Greek mythology, fairy tales, classical and contemporary literature, and today's television. Dr. Ransohoff puts these myths into four basic categories:

The voracious woman. This term does not refer to a heavy eater. Instead, it describes a woman who is sexually greedy and insatiable. In Greek mythology, older women were often depicted as sex-hungry creatures who would turn themselves into beautiful maidens to fulfill their desire. In fairy tales and stories from the Middle Ages, older women were portrayed as sexually aggressive and repulsive, often spending much of their time in orgies and obscene rituals. Even Joan Collins's sexy television character, Alexis Carrington in *Dynasty*, is overdrawn and considered evil. In all cases, these women are eventually made powerless or punished for their sexual desires.

The warlike woman. The familiar image of the older woman as a battle-ax probably comes to mind. From ancient literature to current *Playboy* cartoons, this older woman is so powerful that she has control over life and death. She has a propensity for violence toward men and is often characterized as a control freak—only she knows the answer to the fairy tale riddle that will save the king. In the modern version, she rules the roost, much to the chagrin of her supposedly henpecked mate.

The asexual grandmotherly woman. This woman may seem contradictory to her "voracious" sister, but her image is a common theme when referring to older women. Although she represents a positive, maternal image, she is passive and waits patiently until needed. She imparts wisdom to the next generation and, Dr. Ransohoff says, "is the mother we celebrate on Mother's Day, a woman not without power in her family, but a totally postsexual being." This woman has sworn off sex and sexuality for life—flannel nightgowns only, not a black negligee or red teddy in sight.

The over-the-hill woman. Undoubtedly your worst nightmare, this older woman is seen as physically unappealing, ready for decay, and sexually repugnant. She is a clear representation of death and a reflection of the male fear of physical decline.

What a picture! It is incomprehensible that today's middle-aged women will not have a major impact on changing this image. Take a few who are in the public eye—Jane Fonda, Barbara Jordan, Elizabeth Taylor, Elizabeth Dole, Gloria Steinem—and you are almost forced to rethink what turning 50 actually means.

Moreover, when you think about the social history of women entering midlife today, it is hard to imagine them passively accepting the timeworn image middle age has conjured up. This woman's feelings are typical of many of her peers'.

We may be middle-aged, but we certainly don't think or act the way our parents or grandparents did at that age. I remember when my grandmother was 55. She walked around in this frumpy dress with old lady shoes, her hair done up in a bun. She was actually a demure, proper lady with an elegant demeanor. Yet today, we would describe her as a dumpy old hag. It's a shame to talk about my grandmother that way—mentally she was alert and very with-it for her day—but physically she was old, old, old. She was typical of women at the time—no exercise, no activity, very self-contained attitude. Maybe it's the attitude that's different today, but our version of middle age is radically different. We're more health conscious, interested in physical fitness, and obsessed with our appearance. Our mental and physical attitudes are much younger than my grandmother's, and I truly believe that we're breaking the mold. We're actually redefining middle age. And at this rate, the concepts of old age are just going to be blown to smithereens.

Single mother, 45

Not to be left behind, cosmetics companies are starting to catch on to this potential new image, albeit in a convoluted way.

They still believe looking young is what counts, but they now think that women want to fix certain physical attributes that have broken down with age and perhaps be more in control. These companies have exchanged their former marketing strategy that stressed "hiding" all your wrinkles and defects for one that emphasizes repair and rejuvenation. As examples, Estée Lauder's Advanced Night Repair is effective "in helping skin recover from the effects of daily environmental exposure," and Elizabeth Arden's Ceramide Time Complex Capsules claim to "fix, replenish, or repair the barrier function of the skin."

Alas, they do not quite get it. According to a comment by Kim Gandy of the National Organization for Women that appeared in a *Wall Street Journal* article on cosmetics firms, "Now it's not just 'use this if you want to look beautiful.' It's 'use this or you'll stay broken.'"

Not surprisingly, the marketers most hip to today's middle-aged women are the drug companies that dispense menopause-related products and athletic companies that sell walking shoes. Ciba Pharmaceutical Company, manufacturer of the Estraderm patch, uses the tag line "Now the change of life doesn't have to change yours" on all its promotional material. Nike starts its four-page ad for women's products with a picture of a smiling 12-year-old girl with freckles and pigtails with the caption: "This is a picture of a 40-year-old woman, or perhaps just a picture of the way a 40-year-old woman feels. She is a woman who does not feel her age, or think her age, or act however it is her age is supposed to act."

This is really the heart of the matter. For generations, middle-aged women (and men) have felt young for their years while trapped in an older body. Today's women, with the help of science and their own self-discipline and determination, are making their bodies conform to the way they feel inside. At one extreme is ongoing cosmetic surgery to maintain a youthful appearance, and at another is dedicated physical fitness and diet programs to keep the machine running at peak condition. The goal is the same—to somehow not be a stranger in your own skin.

How Women Feel About Aging

Overall, midlife women are not thrilled with the aging process. Who would be, with an American attitude toward aging women somewhere between indifference and disparagement? Some middle-aged women are devastated by changes in their appearance, whereas others have issues related to work and social acceptance. Yet there are an increasing number of postmenopausal women who not only cope well with the challenge of middle age, but who also go on to new levels of personal development in their 50s and 60s. Clearly, middle age is not the end of the world.

Keeping Up Appearances

> What is beautiful is good, and who is good will soon be beautiful.
> —Sappho, circa 610 B.C.

Try as you may to hold that thought, it can be difficult for a woman to avoid letting a sizable portion of her identity get tied up with her looks. There is nothing more momentous than the first time you look in the mirror and realize that you truly do not look young anymore. Of course, society's obsession with youthful-looking women is enough to make any midlife woman self-conscious, but it is still possible to age gracefully without trying to look like an ingenue. Increased focus on your inner self is an important aspect of aging well, according to this lovely 80-year-old woman who easily maintains grace and charm.

Today's middle-aged women are far too worried about their outward appearance. They focus on changing their bodies in all different ways—breast implants, eye lifts, tummy tucks—and don't value their inner selves. I feel sorry for them, especially when they're convinced that they will no longer be attractive. Of course, not everyone grows old gracefully. And it's hard when you see the wrinkles appear faster and faster. Mentally or emotionally you don't feel that old, but the evidence in the mirror probably tells you otherwise. Your hair gets thinner, everything droops a little more—it can be a very painful time for a woman. To make matters worse, it seems that society has gotten more rigid in its views, with the ideal woman looking younger and younger and younger.

Single woman, 80

On the other hand, many women in their 50s let out a long sigh of relief that they no longer have to try to look like women their daughter's age. After all, emulating model Pauline Porizkova is a lost cause after you turn 40. This woman puts value on her years of experience with her own body and has a rather pragmatic outlook on what is important at this point in the game.

Being middle-aged does have its pluses. After all these years, I've found three styles that hide my figure problems. Each year I load up on what I know looks good and covers all the bad parts. This works well for the office, but I still struggle with sports clothes. My solution? When I take aerobics I don't watch myself in the mirror. I focus on the teacher so I don't have to look at my bouncing breasts or sagging stomach. I guess as an alternative I could go to South America for cosmetic surgery, but it's not my first priority. Getting my daughter into the college of her choice and being able to pay for it is much higher on my list.

Single mother, 52

Disappear down the Rabbit Hole

One of the most startling revelations about midlife is that some women feel they simply become invisible at or around the age of 50. They often categorize this phenomenon as a sort of tuning out of their existence by the rest of the world. An especially dynamic woman described her disappearing act as follows:

When I turned 50, a friend said to me, "Have you noticed that women become invisible at 50?" "What?" I said. "Are you kidding? I'm hardly an invisible person. My hair is about an inch long in bright red—not easy to avoid notice." I told her this notion of invisibility was absurd. But when I started going back to the bar where both my husband and I hang out and dance, I suddenly felt I was invisible—just like my friend had predicted.

It seems like once you're 50, something shuts down in the way society views you. Men don't ask you to dance. Suddenly waitresses begin talking to you as if you're a senior citizen, in sort of a loud tone of voice. It was almost imperceptible at first, but after a year, it was clear that I had become invisible. I looked the same and probably smelled the same, too. But I no longer commanded the authority or exuded the presence that I did when I was 49. And I was totally unprepared.

Married mother, 60

In truth, this woman hardly became invisible. What disappeared was her previous image. Most likely, small changes in her personality and differing ways of relating to people had evolved over the past few years. Certainly people were treating her differently but probably had been doing so for a while without her noticing.

This issue of invisibility is not a silly notion. Carolyn Heilbrun, a well-known author of books about women and the Avalon Foundation Professor of the Humanities at Columbia University in New York City, views this interval of invisibility as a transition period. She feels it spans the time between when a woman, in her youth, is known by how she looks or who looks at her and when a woman, usually in middle age, is known by what she does. In her article "Coming of Age," which appeared in *New York Woman* in 1991, Ms. Heilbrun says, "As older women we will have to be what we do; we will watch ourselves grow invisible to youth worshipers, and to the male gaze. Despair is inevitable but must be wrestled with. The hardest initiation lies ahead, an initiation as in a fairy tale, readying one for a quest: To get to that new place, a woman must pass through the stage of invisibility."

Being caught unaware and having invisibility creep up from

behind to get you is often the result of not being in tune with getting older and it can make you feel devastated. In order to prevent her disappearance at age 50, this woman focused on being proactive about making things happen in her life. What really made a difference was her focus on the good times to come. She did not define herself by previous accomplishments and experiences. Instead, she had an eye to the future and was open to the opportunities it might hold.

> When I turned 50 three years ago, I had a lot of things happening in my life, most of which were positive. I feel that you always need to have something to look forward to, and if it doesn't exist, create it. At 50, I didn't think that my life was half over. Instead I looked at what I was going to be doing that summer. I guess I have a different perspective. I think it's nuts for people to look at you differently just because you turn 50 or become menopausal. After all, people don't change much, not in a year and certainly not overnight.
>
> Married mother, 53

This forward-looking approach sounds logical and appealing but, in reality, can be difficult to achieve. If you view the feeling of invisibility as a transition period, it is often easier to handle. According to Ms. Heilbrun, "We will move invisibly for a time, to relearn seeing and forget being seen. Our voices will ramify, our bodies will become the house for our new spirit."

Coping with and Accepting Middle Age

Aging is relentless, and it is not going to go away anytime soon. By now, you have probably figured out that you have choices about how you respond to its profound effects on your life. The more positive-thinking women, like this one, will find some way to eke out the benefits of midlife without becoming depressed by the downside of the aging process.

> I'd like to think that now that I'm middle-aged, I'm a lot wiser. By now, I've grown up for the most part and have all my values

firmly in place—the things that are most important, priorities, perspective. It's not like I have all the answers, but I definitely have most of them. I've worked out the major kinks in my life, am more sensitive and aware, and have a better understanding of people and of myself.

Married woman, 48

Letting go of previous hangups and relinquishing unreachable goals are just some of the major benefits of getting older. So, too, are having more time to do what is important and finding new meaningful activities to focus on. Nevertheless, all of these goodies come wrapped in a physically older package. This woman's comments aptly express the catch-22 aspect of middle age.

Middle age is a nice time in one sense. The responsibilities are less, I have time to do the activities I didn't have time for before, and my husband and I do more together now that the children are gone. The difficult part is that nobody wants to get old. I think and feel like a young woman, but I know I can't physically operate the same way anymore, and it's scary and frustrating at the same time. I see the end . . . it isn't forever like I thought it was when I was young. And with my mother dying last year, I feel like I'm next in line. But I manage to cope because I'd rather be here on earth in this state than six feet underground.

Married mother, 55

In addition to confronting your own feelings about getting older, most midlife women come up against the prejudiced views of society in one way or another. The first time you experience out-and-out narrow-mindedness because of your age can be a real shock, and it is usually infuriating. Often, it happens more subtly and can even threaten your livelihood if it happens at work.

An extremely successful executive, this woman continues to hide her age in an effort to avoid discrimination and, more importantly, to ensure the continued respect of her co-workers.

The reason I don't tell anyone at work how old I am is because everybody around here is young. I think if they knew, they would look at me differently and I certainly don't want them to think of me as their mother. I'm their supervisor, not their parent.

Single woman, 58

Yes, women are still lying about their age and not just to fool a likely suitor. For many women who work, it is a matter of self-preservation. Using creative measures, this woman who works in executive training and management development has devised a way to protect herself and still be personal with her fellow workers.

I don't hide the fact of how old I am . . . I just don't talk about it. When I'm running seminars, for instance, I rarely mention my oldest daughter. Sometimes if I have to tell an anecdote or talk about something personal, I'll mention my youngest child. I do it to protect myself. If I talk about my oldest, I don't want to hear "I can't believe you really have a 33-year-old daughter" and then watch them go through the mathematics to figure out how old I am. Right now I'm not treated any differently because of my age, and I want to make sure it continues that way.

Married mother, 53

Recently, I found myself in the situation of being the second-oldest woman in the advertising agency where I worked for several years. I was proud of my position in the firm, and the years of both professional and life experience gave me a high level of confidence in what I was doing. Although the gap of more than a decade that separated me from the majority of other women was daunting, there was a real benefit in having worked in a specific area for a significant amount of time. This woman had a similar experience.

It's not easy having a corporate job and being middle-aged. The financial field, like many others, is very youth oriented in terms of hiring, and working with people my daughter's age makes me feel very old. I would chair a group meeting, and there wouldn't be anyone in the room over 30. But as I moved up in the organiza-

tion, being older had its advantages. Because you're always competing with younger people, you gain more credibility and have more of an inside track.

Single woman, 49

Women in their late 60s and beyond have undoubtedly experienced some form of age discrimination. In many ways, it is just these women who can offer the most help, guidance, and inspiration as you confront the trials of midlife. They have been there and have discovered how to cope. This woman benefits enormously from her relationship with her older friend.

I spent the afternoon with a friend of mine who's 72. She's outrageous! We walked to the theater, went to a show, walked to the museum, and then walked across the park for a late afternoon spot of tea. I loved it! And then I have friends who are really stuck in middle age and are younger than I am. They've gotten heavy, only want to go on cruises, and when you tell them you walked a mile, they look at you like you've lost your mind. It's interesting to see the different directions people decide to take with their lives.

Single woman, 59

Through the Looking Glass

"Who are you?" said the Caterpillar. . . . "I hardly know, Sir, just at present," Alice replied rather shyly, "at least I know who I was when I got up this morning, but I think I must have been changed several times since then."

—Lewis Carroll, *Alice's Adventures in Wonderland*

Even without munching a magic cookie or two, your experience with menopause and middle age usually brings about significant changes in your outlook on life. It is a rare person who claims to be unaffected by this rite of passage. Over and over, midlife women use terms such as *coming out the other side, metamorphosis, rebirth,* and *transformation* to describe their new perspective on the world several years past menopause.

As appealing as the concept of change might be, it is also scary to think of becoming a different person at this stage of the game. Very few people are accustomed to trying new things after they turn 40, and just the thought of being different than you were before can cause anxiety. Yet, if you listen to the experts and to women who have emerged from "the other side," this journey is the one that will bring you happiness and fulfillment.

Having successfully completed her journey, this woman talks about the dangers of fighting the aging process and not being open to new ideas.

> *The aging process is not menopause. Menopause is only part of it. Aging means you eventually lose your hearing, your eyesight, and your memory. And if you don't accept it with some grace and humor and amend your life accordingly, you will end up one unhappy person. What you do by fighting it is trying to hold on to what was rather than create what is possible. By fighting the aging process, you don't even see the new possibilities or look for alternatives. Aging is something you really have to face sooner or later. If you don't, you end up in limbo, probably vacillating between hysteria and depression.*
>
> Married mother, 60

In order to make this life transition, it seems that it is not necessary to do anything more than remain open-minded, with a willingness to change. This is not the time to feel you must control the world. In fact, it is probably better to let daily events unfold as they will under your very observant gaze.

After talking with her older friends, this woman is convinced that this postmenopausal metamorphosis is real and one to be valued, despite the trials and tribulations of midlife.

> *There are certain aspects about menopause that you just have to grin and bear, that can't be controlled 100 percent of the time. Sure, you can do something, but women shouldn't feel guilty about not feeling wonderful all the time. It isn't their fault. Women I have spoken with who are postmenopausal talk about a great rise*

in self-esteem, increased energy levels, and a kind of regrouping and getting on with your life afterward. And it doesn't seem to be anything that you do that brings about this splendid change. After menopause, you don't go back to being the person you were, but you do come out feeling invigorated and pushed forward to do the kinds of things you really want to do.

Single mother, 53

Outlook for the Future

Although older people are still not valued by Western society, they are becoming more and more visible as they live longer, healthier lives. At this point, the term *older* seems appropriate. With continued medical breakthroughs and advanced technology targeted at making daily life easier, the boundaries between what are now considered middle and old age will become even fuzzier. Is a 71-year-old woman who runs 4 miles a day considered to be old? What about a 69-year-old who starts a new business? Perhaps it is just a matter of semantics; after all, what is a number anyway. More important than your sequential age is your biological and mental age.

It is not surprising that today's growing number of active older people living well into their 70s and 80s are in the limelight. Even with this shift of attention, it is difficult to project whether the American culture will ever revere older people. However, every day, in growing numbers, they are making their mark on the world.

What will life be like for you at 67 or 77 or 84 years? It is almost impossible to imagine, unless you are lucky enough to have older friends or are privy to the lives of older women. These days, it seems as though almost anything is possible.

The Melpomene Institute, a national organization based in Minneapolis, dedicated to helping women of all ages link physical activity and health through research, publications, and education, published several profiles of older women in its summer 1992 issue of the *Melpomene Journal*. These in-depth and extremely personal autobiographical articles were enlightening about what the future may hold for many of us.

In one of these articles, Edith Mucke, alive since the beginning of World War I, muses about retiring from her position as director of continuing education for women at the University of Minnesota.

I faced my "graduation from the world of work outside the home for pay" with a great deal of ambivalence. I grieved for all the good of the past twenty years and feared the lack of structure, the loss of social and intellectual companionship integral to my daily life there. Yet, I knew I did not want to work another year. I wanted to spend time with my retired husband and sensed that at 69 it was time for me to leave.

How would I face the transition? Would the long list of things I'd been planning and hoping to do in the distant future—when I'd be allowed the luxury of deciding how to spend each day—be as intriguing as it had seemed at an earlier time? Or would I give in to gravity and inertia, and put comfort and lack of stress on the top of the list? How would I fill that wide and deep abyss of time?

After her husband's death six years later, Edith went through another powerful transition.

I was 75, and I knew something about the grieving experience. After all, hadn't I lost my youth, my parents, my middle age, my "work outside the home for pay," the resilience of a 50-year-old body, and so on and so on? Life is a grim series of losses.

As part of the healing process, Edith accepted that there is a reason to be alive and it is not essential to know why. At 77, she came to believe that she was here to learn and took stock of her knowledge.

I've learned that I'm not invulnerable. I've learned that a strong, healthy body is nothing to take for granted. I've learned to appreciate my good genes, a happy mother and a loving family that reinforced what I believe to be an inherently positive attitude toward life.

I listen to my body. If I can't walk all the way around Lake Harriet every single day, I can walk partway every day—or I can walk all the way around every other day.

I must take care of my body if I'm to enjoy old age. I don't have to get old and sick to die. I can simply get old and die.

Edith learned about many things including the dangers of self-denial, the virtue of patience, the reward of no longer being single-minded. Her description of growing older is almost seductive.

Time is a spiral. We meet the past in the present; the past melds with the present.

I look forward. I read. I teach. I write. Every day will bring me gifts—sometimes surprise gifts: a letter from a child or grandchild or friend, a phone call, the first lilies of the valley. A bridge hand may even fan out to a 26 count.

I lead. I follow. I share.

Although Edith and her contemporaries are well past menopause, they are still growing and changing. Their stories are more about daily victories and satisfaction than about headline-grabbing achievements. Given their experiences, it seems that the transition you make after menopause is just the groundwork for moving gracefully through the many changes and challenges that lie ahead.

Appendix 1

Seven Points Every Man Should Know About Menopause

Menopause? I know my wife goes through a lot of hormonal stuff, but I get it all confused with postmenstrual syndrome. It's as clearly defined to me as a man's midlife crisis.

Married father, 58

This section is for men. It will take about ten minutes to read and will provide you with enough basics about menopause so that you will be able to talk about it, if called on to do so, with your mate or other women. Reading this will not make you an expert but will definitely put you ahead of most other men. It will also raise your stock with the women in your life.

1. Menopause Is Real

Of course, women stop menstruating around the age of 51 and can no longer become pregnant—that is a cold, hard fact. However, the chemistry behind this reality also sets the stage for other less familiar menopausal indicators that are just as real.

As a woman ages, she uses up most of her eggs, and the remaining ones become dysfunctional. This leads to decreased production of various hormones by the ovaries, especially estrogen, until finally, at the age of 51—give or take a few years—menstruation stops entirely. It is this gradual decrease in estrogen that begins in a woman's early to mid-40s that may bring on many of the signs of menopause like fragmented sleep, hot flashes, night sweats, vaginal dryness, loss of libido, unpredictable or heavy bleeding, urinary stress incontinence, and mood swings. This is a normal, natural occurrence experienced by all women to one degree or another.

Just as no two individuals are alike, no two women go through menopause in the same way. There is no such thing as "a typical menopause," and heredity does not play much of a role. Furthermore, women are unable to readily control how their bodies respond to decreasing hormones. As a result of menopausal changes, their mood swings and bodily changes may surprise them just as much as they do you.

The important point to keep in mind is that women experience a variety of uncontrollable body changes related to menopause, all of which are legitimate and deserve recognition.

2. Menopause Is a Transition

Similar to adolescence, menopause is a time of physical and emotional change. It is a major event that represents the transition between a woman's childbearing years and the second half of her life. According to Gail Sheehy, author of *The Silent Passage* (New York: Random House, 1992), "If forty-five is the old age of youth, fifty is the youth of Second Adulthood."

Like most transitions, menopause is a temporary period of ups and downs that often challenges a woman's patience and equilibrium. For some, the transition can last a couple of years, and for others, it can take from six to ten years. During this time, women may feel less sure of themselves and often question the very things that previously gave them comfort and security. For them, menopause is a very real sign that they are passing into a new and unfamiliar phase of life. In addition to the physical signs of menopause, they are concerned about issues such as

- Life without children at home.
- Effects of getting older.
- Satisfaction with work and other outside interests.
- Continued sexual attractiveness.
- Aging, ailing parents and in-laws.

You will find that women respond to menopause in much the same way they have to other physical and emotional problems. In the end, most women appear much the same but with the addition of a stronger sense of self-confidence and a positive outlook on the future.

3. Menopause May Cause You to Lose Sleep

You always thought you were a sympathetic kind of guy, but did you ever think you would be up all night because of menopause? You may be one of the lucky few who regularly sleep with a menopausal woman and snooze blissfully through the night. The remaining majority will find their sleep disturbed by a new wrinkle in the bid-for-the-blanket war—menopausal night sweats or hot flashes.

Experienced by 80 percent of all women, hot flashes are amazing events in which a woman's body temperature actually increases by as much as 7 degrees, her pulse speeds up, and she invariably breaks out in a sweat. All of this can happen while just sitting still, walking around the block, or peacefully sleeping. Hot flashes usually last a few minutes, and only 10 to 15 percent of women find them debilitating. Most women will experience them at some level for more than a year, yet merely 25 percent will continue to have them for more than five years.

Although not completely certain, scientists believe hot flashes occur when a woman's body temperature control center, located in the hypothalamus, becomes imbalanced. Once this thermostat is affected—probably as a result of hormonal fluctuation—the ability to adjust body temperature is thrown off. The result: a hot flash by day or night sweats when the lights are out.

Where does this leave you? Either fighting for the covers to keep warm or at your local bedding store about to purchase a dual-control electric blanket.

At first, hot flashes can be novel and amusing. However, as they continue and perhaps keep one or both of you up at night, the humor can wear thin. This can mean continual feelings of exhaustion, crankiness on both your parts, and frustration about lack of control. Fortunately, hot flashes eventually stop. Until then you might want to pay attention to ongoing research, some of which suggests that warm temperatures can trigger night sweats. Help your mate by keeping the bedroom cool. You also might want to think about buying a down comforter for your side of the bed.

4. Menopause Can Influence Your Sex Life

Sex with a menopausal woman can go either way: It can get better than you ever dreamed or stop almost entirely.

With the end of menstruation comes the beginning of sex without contraception. This can be terrific for both partners, and as a result, some women become liberated and more adventurous in bed. No longer having children in the house can also lead to more fun and games. In fact, many men wish the timetable had been reversed now that they find themselves living with a more interested and passionate lover.

With the pendulum swinging the other way, a formerly healthy sex life can be plagued by the effects of vaginal dryness, namely, painful sex for your mate. A woman's vagina, usually very elastic with incredible stretching ability, starts to shrink as available estrogen decreases. It becomes thinner, easier to tear, and loses some of its mucous membrane. As drastic as these changes may sound, they can be reversed with regular sexual activity—once a week will do the trick. The issues, though, are how to have sex if it hurts and, for men in particular, how to know when your tenderness and affection is actually causing pain and discomfort.

Another menopausal indicator that can put a crimp in your sex life is a lack of interest on the part of your mate. The loss of libido may be experienced by some women and is not necessarily a reflection on you and your sexual attractiveness. Like most emotions, libido is affected by a combination of factors working together: sex hormones, psyche, environment, and the sexual partner. This condition is often temporary, and if you and your partner both have an interest in an active sex life, flagging libido can be dealt with and overcome.

Perhaps the simplest way to cope with changes in your sex life is to talk about them. This may be a new strategy for you, but you will find it to be well worth the effort. There is no reason to assume that menopause means the end of your sex life. In fact, it may be just the kind of catalyst you need to discover new kinds of pleasure with your mate.

5. All of the Above May Affect a Woman's Disposition

Contrary to popular rumors, menopause does not cause depression or lunacy, nor does it mean that your mate's personality will never be the same again. Studies show that women who have recently gone through menopause did not have higher levels of depression, anxiety, or stress than women of the same age who were still menstruating.

Nevertheless, menopause does bring on definite chemical changes in a woman's body, some of which may result in a more heightened premenstrual syndrome, for a week or so each month. Mood swings that may occur subsequently are not a fabrication, and it is difficult for many women to control them. Furthermore, menopause happens at about the same time women experience a myriad of other changes mentioned earlier. If you combine all these factors, you are bound to see a deviation from a woman's normal emotional profile. After all, how would you feel in this kind of situation?

Keep in mind, none of these changes is permanent. However, you may have to cope with a woman's variable disposition for several years until the effects of menopause and other life events become less volatile.

6. FYI

Below is a list of issues associated with menopause that are of great concern to women. Although you may not become actively involved in working through answers tied to these issues, it is important for you to know about their existence.

Heart Disease

The number one cause of death in women, heart disease becomes even more threatening after menopause. In a single year, out of 2,000 post-menopausal women, 20 will get heart disease and 12 will die from it.

There is no question that postmenopausal women are at a significantly higher risk of cardiovascular disease than their premenopausal counterparts. After menopause, lack of estrogen causes the ratio of good cholesterol to bad cholesterol to shift dramatically, usually within six months after menstruation has stopped. This results in an increased overall cholesterol level for the postmenopausal woman and, more significantly, a level that has a higher proportion of bad cholesterol.

To combat this increased risk, women are looking at revised eating habits, new exercise regimes, no smoking, less drinking, and hormone replacement therapy.

Osteoporosis

One out of every four postmenopausal women will develop osteoporosis, increasing their risk for spinal and hip fractures as well as other debilitating conditions. Once people with osteoporosis sustain a fracture, their quality of life is severely compromised and they often spend the rest of their days in pain and discomfort.

How does menopause figure into this picture? Basically all humans lose bone mass as they age, but for eight to ten years after menopause, a woman's lack of estrogen accelerates the process, and she can lose as much as 3 to 6 percent each year.

Because a cure for osteoporosis has yet to be discovered, the emphasis is on prevention. This means a woman needs to concentrate her efforts on the following measures: a diet rich in calcium, calcium supplements if necessary, weight-bearing exercise to increase bone mass, regular monitoring of bone mass density, and the option of hormone replacement therapy.

Hormone Replacement Therapy

The single biggest controversy associated with menopause is whether or not a woman should take hormone replacement therapy. This is not simply a matter of indecision. There has just not been enough long-term research done in this area to assure women that taking hormones is free from risk.

Some studies have shown that estrogen, taken alone, can decrease the risk of heart disease by 40 to 60 percent. Other studies indicate that if estrogen is taken with progesterone—necessary to prevent endometrial cancer in women who still have a uterus—this positive effect on heart disease risk may be reversed.

On the other hand, estrogen, with or without progesterone, has been proven to have a beneficial effect on retarding osteoporotic bone loss. Yet long-term use of estrogen may moderately increase the risk of breast cancer.

With the available data, women must now make their decision

based on a numbers game. They are faced with statistics like the following from which they must try to determine their need for hormone replacement therapy and make a decision.

Women over 50 have a

31   percent risk of dying from heart disease.
2.8 percent risk of dying from breast cancer.
2.8 percent risk of a hip fracture.
0.7 percent risk of endometrial cancer.

Looking at these same issues from another perspective, for every 2,000 postmenopausal women

20 will develop heart disease.
 6 will develop breast cancer.
11 will develop severe bone loss.
 3 will develop endometrial cancer.

This is the dilemma women face every day whether they are pre- or postmenopausal. Their alternatives to hormone replacement therapy center around altered diet, exercise programs, vitamins, herbs, and other forms of natural medicine—many of which have proven helpful to a certain degree. Unfortunately, the uncertainty around the long-term use of hormone replacement therapy will exist for at least another ten years, until longitudinal studies have been completed.

7. What You Can Do to Help

Simply put, men just need to be there for women during menopause. This is a tough time for women because of the uncertainty of how they will experience menopause and subsequent feelings of loss of control of their body. It really is not much fun.

Men can have a major positive influence by being even-tempered and supportive. Your mate may not be able to articulate much of what is happening to her or perhaps will not want to talk about it at all. However, she will still want your comfort and has a high need to know you truly care and still find her attractive. As a man, you have a great deal of power to make a difference for a woman going through menopause.

Appendix 2

Resources

The resources listed here are personal favorites. They are arranged by subject interest and should be helpful in your quest for additional information. Be aware that there are many more resources available, with new publications coming out on a regular basis. So use this list as a starting point and keep your eyes open for others.

Menopause

Books

Budoff, Penny Wise, M.D., *No More Hot Flashes* (New York: Warner Books, 1984).
  Although this book has been around for quite some time, Dr. Budoff's technical explanations of various body changes related to menopause are extremely helpful to women who want more detail. The majority of information is still up-to-date.

Cutler, Winnifred B., Ph.D., and Celso-Ramon Garcia, M.D., *Menopause, A Guide for Women and the Men Who Love Them*, Rev. Ed. (New York: W. W. Norton & Company, 1992).
  Well researched, this somewhat technical book will provide the average woman with a scholarly knowledge of menopause. What it may lack in warmth and readability, it makes up for in accurate, detailed information.

Greenwood, Sadja, M.D., *Menopause Naturally*, Rev. Ed. (Volcano, CA: Volcano Press, 1989).

Easy to read, this book presents both sides of the hormone replacement therapy question and briefly discusses the complete range of other menopause-related issues.

Henig, Robin Marantz, *How a Woman Ages* (New York: Ballantine Books, 1985).
Although this book is not exclusively about menopause, it covers many midlife issues and helps put the menopause experience in perspective. In practical and nonemotional terms, it presents a clear picture of what physical changes to expect with aging.

Lark, Susan M., M.D., *The Menopause Self-Help Book* (Berkeley, CA: Celestial Arts, 1990).
This book focuses on alternative ways to deal with signs of menopause, from diet and exercise to vitamins, herbs, and acupressure massage. It is well written, and specific remedies are recommended for individual problems.

Nachtigall, Lila E., and Joan Rattner Heilman, *Estrogen*, Rev. Ed. (New York: HarperCollins, 1991).
Dr. Nachtigall presents the benefits and risks of hormone replacement therapy in a fairly balanced fashion. This is a useful, readable book for women who want to learn up-to-date information about hormone replacement therapy to help with decision making.

Ojeda, Linda, Ph.D., *Menopause Without Medicine*, Rev. Ed. (Alameda, CA: Hunter House, 1992).
A no-nonsense approach to coping with menopause, Dr. Ojeda's book offers natural strategies and solutions, with emphasis on nutrition and exercise.

Wolfe, Honora Lee, *Second Spring, A Guide to Healthy Menopause Through Traditional Chinese Medicine*, 2d ed. (Boulder, CO: Blue Poppy Press, 1992).
In addition to providing an alternative to orthodox treatments of menopause, this book is an excellent primer on the theories of traditional Chinese medicine. It is clearly written and easy to understand, even if you have no background in Chinese medicine. However, information on estrogen is dated and you will need to consult other sources.

Newsletters

A Friend Indeed, Janine O'Leary Cobb, founder and editor. Published monthly, except July and August. Write Box 515, Place du Parc Station, Montreal, Canada H2W 2P1, (514) 843-5730.

An informative, unbiased publication, *A Friend Indeed* tackles difficult menopause issues on a regular basis. Nearly half of every issue is dedicated to a readers' exchange, where women write in about problems and share their experiences.

Hot Flash: A Newsletter for Midlife and Older Women, Dr. Jane Porcino, editor-in-chief. Published quarterly by the National Action Forum for Midlife and Older Women, Box 816, Stony Brook, NY 11790-0609.

This newsletter covers a wide variety of social and health issues relevant to midlife and older women.

Menopause News, Judith S. Askew, publisher. Published six times a year by Menopause News, 2074 Union Street, San Francisco, CA 94123, (415) 567-2368.

Relatively new, this newsletter has become more technically thorough with each published issue. It covers a wide range of midlife topics including menopause in general, aging, the latest on available drug treatment, and spiritual issues. Letters to the editors are published regularly and books of interest to midlife women are reviewed in each publication.

Midlife Woman, Sharon Slettehaugh, publisher; Carole Moore, editor. Published bimonthly (six issues a year) by Midlife Women's Network, 5129 Logan Avenue South, Minneapolis, MN 55419, (612) 925-0020.

This new newsletter regularly covers the topic of menopause and also focuses on other issues related to midlife women such as successful aging, widowhood, sexuality, and self-esteem. Its viewpoint is current and represents the trend to redefine middle age.

Organizations

American College of Obstetricians and Gynecologists, Office of Public Information, 409 12th Street SW, Washington, DC 20024-2188, (202) 484-3321.

Homeopathic Educational Services, 2124 Kittredge Street, Berkeley, CA 94704, (510) 649-0294.

This organization is an excellent source of homeopathic books, tapes, medicines, software, and general information.

National Center for Homeopathy, 810 North Fairfax, Suite 306, Alexandria, VA 22314, (703) 548-7790.
This organization coordinates the activities of over one hundred homeopathy study groups throughout the country and will provide you with the name of one in your area.

National Women's Health Network, 1325 G Street NW, Washington, DC 20005, (202) 347-1140.
The only national organization devoted solely to women and health, this organization represents over 500,000 women and accepts no financial support from pharmaceutical companies. Its position paper on hormone replacement therapy is comprehensive and will be useful to any woman seeking information about use of these drugs and menopause.

North American Menopause Society, Wulf H. Utian, M.D., Ph.D., president, University Hospitals Department of OB/GYN, 2074 Abington Road, Cleveland, OH 44106, (216) 844-3334.
Founded in 1989, this multidisciplinary organization will provide a list of menopause clinics in your area as well as names of local physicians.

Audiotapes

Northrup, Christiane, M.D., *Honoring Our Bodies, Reclaiming Women's Wisdom*. Produced by Women to Women, 1 Pleasant Street, Yarmouth, ME 04096, (207) 846-6163.
An entertaining and informative lecturer, Dr. Northrup shares her experiences with patients and her own viewpoints on menopause, hormone replacement therapy, and societal attitudes toward midlife women. She feels menopause is a natural phenomenon and places a strong emphasis on women taking charge of their own bodies and health care.

Women's Midlife Health Project, *Myths and Realities about Menopause*. GPA, 74 Witch Tree Road, Woodstock, NY 12498, (914) 679-7890.
A series of six lectures on hormone replacement therapy, alternative treatments, sexuality, psychology, and preventive health care.

Heart Disease

Books

Legato, Marianne, M.D., and Carol Colman, *The Female Heart: The Truth About Women and Coronary Artery Disease* (New York: Simon & Schuster, 1991).

Natural Progesterone

Natural progesterone is available only with a doctor's prescription.

Belmar Pharmacy in Lakewood, CO, is an excellent source of natural progesterone, estradiol, and testosterone in hypoallergenic tablets: (800) 525-9473.

Madison Pharmacy Associates and PMS Access in Madison, WI, have a fifteen-year track record of compounding natural progesterone in tablet, suppository, and sublingual forms: (800) 222-4767.

Nutrition and Exercise

Books

Connor, Sonja L., M.S., R.D., and William E. Connor, M.D., *The New American Diet System* (New York: Simon & Schuster, 1991).
This is an easy-to-understand book on good nutrition, complete with calorie, fat, and carbohydrate counts on almost every food under the sun. Their Cholesterol–Saturated Fat Index (CSI) helps you quickly determine the food that is healthiest.

Melpomene Institute for Women's Health Research, *The Bodywise Woman* (New York: Prentice Hall Press, 1990).
Written by researchers and staff at Melpomene, this book was put together by women for women. It focuses on sensible ways to remain active throughout your life and addresses many issues related to fitness and aging.

Ornish, Dean, M.D., *Dr. Dean Ornish's Program for Reversing Heart Disease* (New York: Ballantine Books, 1990).

This book is not just for heart patients. It is for anyone who has a serious interest in keeping her body in good shape through diet and exercise. Dr. Ornish makes it easy to learn how to take steps to control your long-term good health.

Newsletters

Nutrition Action Healthletter, Michael F. Jacobson, Ph.D., executive director; Stephen B. Schmidt, editor. Published ten times a year by the Center for Science in the Public Interest, Suite 300, 1875 Connecticut Avenue NW, Washington, DC 20009-5728.

At the forefront of consumer education, this publication provides up-to-the-minute information about such topics as healthy alternatives to fast food, health food hoaxes, twenty-minute meals, and foods that lower blood pressure and reduce the risk of breast cancer.

Tufts University Diet & Nutrition Letter, Stanley N. Gershoff, Ph.D., dean, School of Nutrition, editor. Published monthly by Tufts University Diet and Nutrition Letter, 53 Park Place, New York, NY 10007. Write Box 57857, Boulder, CO 80322-7857, for new subscription information.

Filled with informative, up-to-date information written for laypeople, this newsletter addresses issues important to everyone, whether or not they are saintly eaters.

Special Organizations, Publications, and Services

Melpomene [mel•POM•uh•nee], *A Journal for Women's Health Research*, Judy Mahle Lutter, president; Judy Remington, editor. Published three times a year by the Melpomene Institute, 1010 University Avenue, St. Paul, MN 55104, (612) 642-1951.

Named for the woman runner who scandalized the 1896 Olympics by illegally running in the marathon, the Melpomene Institute is a nonprofit organization that helps women of all ages link physical activity and health through its research, publications, and education. Information packets are available on a wide range of topics from menopause, osteoporosis, and PMS to fitness walking and aging well. This is a down-to-earth organization that most women, whether athletic or hoping to be, will identify with quite easily.

Nutritive Value of Foods, Home and Garden Bulletin No. 72. Published by the Superintendent of Documents, U.S. Government Printing Office, Washington, DC 20402.

This handy, inexpensive booklet from the U.S. Department of Agriculture gives nutrition information for more than 900 foods, including numbers for calories, protein, fats, sodium, cholesterol, carbohydrates, iron, calcium, and several vitamins.

What's in It? The Busy Cook's Diet and Nutrition Guides. Published by Nutrifino, 825 University Avenue, Norwood, MA 02062, (800) 676-6686.

Fifteen guides to the cookbooks listed below provide per-serving values for the calories, fat, saturated fat, sodium, cholesterol, carbohydrates, and protein in every recipe.

Chef Paul Prudhomme's Louisiana Kitchen
The Classic Italian Cookbook
Crockery Cookery
The Enchanted Broccoli Forest Cookbook
The Fannie Farmer Cookbook
The Frugal Gourmet
The Frugal Gourmet Cooks with Wine
The Moosewood Cookbook
Microwave Gourmet
The New Basics Cookbook
The New York Times Cookbook
The New York Times 60-Minute Gourmet
The Silver Palate Cookbook
The Silver Palate Good Times Cookbook
The Way to Cook

Osteoporosis

Books

Peck, William A., M.D., and Louis V. Avioli, M.D., *Osteoporosis— The Silent Thief* (Glenview, IL: AARP Books, 1988).

Organizations

National Osteoporosis Foundation, Sandra C. Raymond, executive director, 1150 17th Street NW, Suite 500, Washington, DC 20036, (800) 223-9994 or (202) 223-2226.

Founded in 1984, the National Osteoporosis Foundation (NOF) is the only nonprofit, voluntary health agency wholly dedicated to the prevention and treatment of osteoporosis. In addition to promoting research and conducting medical and scientific conferences, the NOF encourages public awareness through publication of a wide variety of excellent educational booklets, such as *Boning Up on Osteoporosis, A Guide to Prevention and Treatment; Stand Up to Osteoporosis;* and *The Older Person's Guide to Osteoporosis.* They also publish a quarterly newsletter entitled *The Osteoporosis Report.* The NOF is the key advocacy group for those interested in changing attitudes and legislation related to osteoporosis.

Psychological, Emotional, and Spiritual Growth

Books

Estes, Clarissa Pinkola, Ph.D., *Women Who Run with the Wolves* (New York: Ballantine Books, 1992).
   A book about women recovering the creative, passionate soul force within—one too often masked by societal roles and expectations. Jean Shinoda Bolen, M.D., describes it as "full of wonderful, passionate, poetic, psychologically potent words and images that will inspire, instruct, and empower women to be true to their own nature, and thus in touch with sources of creativity, humor, and strength."

Sanford, Linda Tschirhart, and Mary Ellen Donovan, *Women and Self-Esteem: Understanding and Improving the Way We Think and Feel About Ourselves* (New York: Penguin Books, 1984).
   A helpful resource for women in building self-esteem, this book examines the cultural, media, and religious institutions that shape women's negative attitudes about themselves. It offers a broad perspective to help women understand the source of their feelings of inadequacy and insecurity and offers concrete help in the form of exercises to help improve feelings of self-worth.

Walker, Barbara G., *The Crone: Woman of Age, Wisdom, and Power* (San Francisco: Harper & Row, 1985).

This book helps women understand the historical roots of the devaluation, repression, and denial of the wisdom of older women. It also offers insights into ways women may develop the kind of constructive, healing power that will benefit present and future societies.

Sex

Books

Barbach, Lonnie, *For Each Other: Sharing Sexual Intimacy* (New York: Anchor Press/Doubleday, 1982).
A self-help guide for women who can sometimes reach orgasm but want more satisfaction or communication. This book also discusses painful intercourse.

Barbach, Lonnie, *For Yourself: The Fulfillment of Female Sexuality* (New York: Anchor Press/Doubleday, 1975).
This is a self-help guide for women having trouble reaching orgasm.

Heiman, Julia, and Joseph LoPiccolo, *Becoming Orgasmic: A Sexual and Personal Growth Program for Women* (Englewood Cliffs, NJ: Prentice-Hall, 1988).
This book provides comprehensive information on women's sexuality.

Stoppard, Mariam, M.D., *The Magic of Sex: The Book That Really Tells Men About Women and Women About Men* (New York: Dorling Kindersly, Inc., 1991).
This sensitive manual stresses that the most fulfilling sex is found in stable, long-term relationships. Sex is discussed from both the man's and woman's point of view.

Audiotapes

Zilbergeld, Bernie, and Lonnie Barbach, *How to Talk with a Partner About Smart Sex*. The Sexuality Library, 3385 22nd Street, San Francisco, CA 94110.

Special Problems

Books

Burgio, K. L., Ph.D., A. J. Lucco, M.D., and K. L. Pearce, R.N., *Staying Dry, A Practical Guide to Bladder Control.* (Baltimore: Johns Hopkins University Press, 1989).

Cutler, Winnifred B., Ph.D., *Hysterectomy: Before and After* (New York: Harper & Row, 1988).

Dalton, Katharina, M.D., *Once a Month: A Guide to the Effects, Diagnosis, and Treatment of Premenstrual Syndrome* (Claremont, CA: Hunter House, 1986).

Eades, Mary Dan, M.D., *Breast Cancer: If It Runs in Your Family, How to Reduce Your Risk* (New York: Bantam Books, 1991).

Goldfarb, Herbert A., M.D., with Judith Greif, *The No-Hysterectomy Option: Your Body—Your Choice* (New York: John Wiley & Sons, 1990).

Hummel, Sherilynn J., M.D., and Marie Lindquist, *Ovarian and Uterine Cancer: If It Runs in Your Family, Reducing Your Risk* (New York: Bantam Books, 1992).

Special Services

HERS (Hysterectomy Educational Resources and Services) Foundation, 422 Bryn Mawr Avenue, Bala Cynwyd, PA 19004, (215) 667-7757 or (215) 387-6700.

A nonprofit organization, HERS provides information about the alternatives to hysterectomy and coping with the consequences of the surgery. Free one-on-one counseling is offered by experts via telephone. They advise over one hundred women each day, addressing issues such as whether or not you have had a proper evaluation, or who are the best people to see about your condition. In addition to publishing a quarterly newsletter (annual fee $20), HERS offers copies of medical journal articles, makes referrals to doctors, and holds conferences semiannually.

Index

McGuire, William L., 288
McKinley, John B., 310
McKinley, Sonja J., 278
Magnesium, 67–68, 93, 186–87
Male midlife crisis, 310–15
Mammograms, 35, 289
Mansfield, Phyllis Kernoff, Ph.D., 234
Mao Zedong, 175
Marital status, sexual frequency and, 236
Maslow, Katie, 95
Mastectomy, 275
Masters, William, 234
Masturbation, 59
  lubricants for, 239–40
Medicare and Medicaid, 196
Meditation, 190
Melpomene Institute, 356–57
Memory loss, 70–72
Men, 302–22
  information about menopause for, 359–65
  knowledge about menopause of, 305–7
  midlife changes for, 310–18
  sexual attractiveness to, 307–10
  sexual relations with, see Sex
  talking about menopause with, 318–22
  views on menopause of, 303–5
Menstruation
  age of starting, 28
  anatomy of, 41–44
  changing patterns of, 29–30, 46–50
  migraines and, 69
  problems with, 27
  short cycles, 25
Mental illness, 28
Middle age, 343–58
  coping with and accepting, 351–54
Migraine headaches, 69
Milk
  skim, 211
  warm, as sleep aid, 57

Miller, Monica, 196
Minerals
  as alternative remedies, 181–90
  See also Calcium
Monounsaturated fat, 208
Mood swings, 64–68
  alternative treatments for, 180, 191–92
  exercise and, 215
  HRT and, 140
  men's response to, 320, 363
  triggers for, 180
Mucke, Edith, 357–68
Myoma coagulation, 296
Myomectomy, 271, 295

Nachtigall, Lila, 238, 275
National Cancer Institute, 212, 290, 293
National Center for Health Statistics, 269
National Heart, Lung and Blood Institute, 115
National Institutes for Health, 115, 318
National Osteoporosis Foundation, 86
National Women's Health Network, 161
New England Journal of Medicine, 95, 113
Night sweats, 51, 52, 54–57
  men's response to, 320, 361–62
Nike, 347
Nolovadex, see Tamoxifen
Nonoxynol 9, 259
Norplant, 256
North American Menopause Society, 342
Nurses' Health Study, 113, 114
Nutrition, 197–214
  emotional health and, 66–67
  fat and, 206–8
  food groups, 203–6
  heart disease and, 107–10
  how to eat right, 209–14
  osteoporosis and, 79–80, 89
  during pregnancy, 25

Steroids, 80–81, 86
Sunscreen, 118
Support groups, 267
Surgically induced menopause, *see*
    Hysterectomy

Tamoxifen, 127, 275, 290–94
Testosterone, 35
    libido and, 231, 243
    male midlife decline and, 316–18
Tosteson, Anna, 162
Trabecular bone, 77
Transdermal patch, 148–49
Triglycerides, 34
Tubal ligation, 26, 256–57, 265
Tufts University, 201
Tums, 91–92

Ullman, Dana, 194
United States Department of Agri-
    culture (USDA), 203
Urinary stress incontinence, 32,
    61–63
    HRT for, 138
Uterus
    cancer of, *see* Endometrial cancer
    changes in, 227
    fibroids, 294-97
Utian, Wulf H., 264

Vaginal cancer, 36, 289
Vaginal dryness, 31–32, 58–61
    after chemotherapy, 290

estrogen cream for, 149–50
    HRT for, 137–38, 157
    men's concerns about, 319, 362
    reversing, 238–42
    sex and, 226–27, 234
Vaginal smear, 36–37
Vaginal sonography, 37
Vasectomy, 257
Vegetables, 211–12
Vegetarianism, 109–10
Venereal disease, 259
Vertebral abnormalities, 86
Vitamin E, 68, 188–89
Vitamins
    as alternative remedies, 181–92
    in complementary medicine, 168
    emotional health and, 67–68
    osteoporosis and, 89–93
    wrinkles and, 119
Vulvar cancer, 289

Walking, 56, 219
Weg, Ruth, 225
Weight
    control of, 198, 200
    exercise and, 215, 216
    heart disease and, 104–5, 108
    hot flashes and, 53
    osteoporosis and, 79
Wilson, Robert A., 124
Women to Women, 333–34
Wrinkles, 116–20
Wyeth-Ayerst Laboratories, 140